Fast Facts

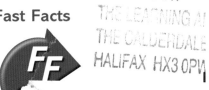

D1388446

r

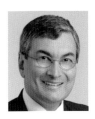

Derek Raghavan MD PhD FACP FRACP
Director and Chair
Cleveland Clinic Taussig Cancer Center
Cleveland, Ohio, USA

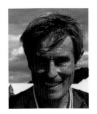

Michael Bailey MS FRCS
Consultant Urologist
St George's Hospital
London, UK

Declaration of Independence

This book is as balanced and as practical as we can
make it. Ideas for improvement are always welcome:
feedback@fastfacts.com

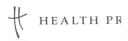

HEALTH PR

Fast Facts: Bladder Cancer
First published 1999
Second edition March 2006

Text © 2006 Derek Raghavan, Michael Bailey
© 2006 in this edition Health Press Limited
Health Press Limited, Elizabeth House, Queen Street, Abingdon,
Oxford OX14 3LN, UK
Tel: +44 (0)1235 523233
Fax: +44 (0)1235 523238

Book orders can be placed by telephone or via the website.
For regional distributors or to order via the website, please go to:
www.fastfacts.com
For telephone orders, please call 01752 202301 (UK), +44 1752 202301 (Europe),
1 800 247 6553 (USA, toll free) or +1 419 281 1802 (Americas).

Fast Facts is a trademark of Health Press Limited.

A CIP record for this title is available from the British Library.

ISBN 1-903734-25-8

Raghavan D (Derek)
Fast Facts: Bladder Cancer/
Derek Raghavan, Michael Bailey

Medical illustrations by Dee McLean, London, UK.
Typesetting and page layout by Zed, Oxford, UK.
Indexed by Laurence Errington, Edinburgh, UK.
Printed by Fine Print (Services) Ltd, Oxford, UK.

Printed with vegetable inks on fully biodegradable and
recyclable paper manufactured from sustainable forests.

444   001
Low emissions
during production

Low
chlorine

Sustainable
forests

Glossary

AMH: asymptomatic microscopic hematuria

Anaplasia: loss of typical cell characteristics or differentiation that can occur, for example, in rapidly growing malignant tumors

BCG: bacillus Calmette–Guérin, a strain of tubercle bacillus that can stimulate an immune response even though it does not cause tuberculosis

BTA stat test: bladder tumor antigen test

BTA TRAK test: test that quantifies bladder tumor antigen

CAP: cyclophosphamide–doxorubicin–cisplatin

CIS: carcinoma in situ, a high-grade, flat, non-invasive malignant change in the urothelium; also known as Tis

CMV: cisplatin–methotrexate–vinblastine

CT: computed tomography

Cystectomy: surgical removal of the bladder

Cystoscopy: examination of the bladder using a cystoscope

Dysplasia: abnormal development of tissues with cellular changes (some of which may connote increased risk of subsequent bladder cancer), including increased nucleus-to-cytoplasm ratio or cellular irregularity, but with normal mitosis

EORTC: European Organisation for Research and Treatment of Cancer

F/FDP: fibrin/fibrinogen degradation products

HA/HAase: hyaluronic acid/hyaluronidase

HPF: high-powered field

IVU: intravenous urogram

KUB: kidneys, ureters and bladder

MRI: magnetic resonance imaging

MVAC: methotrexate–vinblastine–doxorubicin–cisplatin

NMP: nuclear matrix protein

NMP-22 test: test for an NMP that is secreted by some bladder tumors

Primary CIS: carcinoma in situ in the absence of exophytic tumors

RBC: red blood cell

RTOG: Radiation Therapy Oncology Group

Secondary CIS: carcinoma in situ with associated papillary or solid tumors

TCC: transitional cell carcinoma

TNM: tumor–nodes–metastases, a staging system

TURBT: transurethral resection of a bladder tumor

UBC: urinary bladder cancer

Urography: radiographic examination of the kidneys, ureters and bladder with contrast medium (see IVU)

UTI: urinary tract infection

Introduction

Cancer of the urinary bladder (UBC) is a common tumor, and most primary care physicians will see two or three new cases each year. Since many of these patients will have a good prognosis, the number of patients with bladder cancer in the population of every practice will be much larger.

Our aim in this book is to provide the relevant facts regarding bladder cancer clearly and succinctly, so that those caring for these patients can explain their condition and help them through some of the difficult treatment choices they may have to make. It is intended to be a concise guide to clinical practice rather than a comprehensive textbook, although we have tried to include the evidence base for diagnosis and management of UBC together with recent developments in treatment. *Fast Facts – Bladder Cancer* will also be of interest to patients keen to learn more about their condition, and to junior doctors wanting a concise review of bladder cancer.

In this second edition, we have expanded the sections on chemotherapy and radiotherapy, and provided more detail about oncology and palliation. We hope that you will find the book useful.

We thank Mike Sarosdy for his contributions to the first edition, on which this book is based.

Incidence

The incidence of bladder cancer has risen over the past 20 years. Currently, around 54 500 new cases of bladder cancer are diagnosed in the USA each year, and 15 000 cases in the UK. Bladder cancer is the fourth most common cancer in men in the USA and the tenth most common in women. It is one of the most frequent causes of cancer death, accounting for about 10 000 deaths annually in the USA and 5000 in the UK.

The incidence of bladder cancer varies among different patient groups. For example, there is a 3:1 male-to-female ratio, though the prevalence among women appears to be rising. The incidence is higher in elderly populations, with a median age at presentation of 60–65 years. No evidence exists for a familial or inherited pattern among any patient group, although occasional family clusters have been recorded. In black people the incidence is lower than in white people; in Asian races it appears to be intermediate. The lifetime risk of developing bladder cancer is:

- 2.8% for white men
- 0.9% for black men
- 1.0% for white women
- 0.6% for black women.

Five-year survival for both black and white people during the period 1986–92 (60% and 82%, respectively) was significantly better than the equivalent rates for 1974–76 (47% and 74%, respectively; $p < 0.05$). It is not really known why there are substantial ethnic differences in incidence and prognosis, although putative factors include differences in diet and nutritional status, differences in gene expression (especially of enzymes that may metabolize carcinogens) and differential access to healthcare.

Etiology

A number of factors have been implicated in the development of bladder cancer, including environmental and industrial carcinogens (Table 1.1).

Cigarette smoking. Smoking is now recognized as the prime cause of bladder cancer in industrialized countries. Between 60% and 80% of patients with bladder cancer have a history of cigarette smoking; there is a twofold to fivefold increase in the risk of bladder cancer associated with smoking. (Development of cancer lags 10–20 years behind exposure, so current incidence reflects smoking patterns of up to 20–30 years ago.) Smokers have a higher rate of tumor recurrence and a greater proportion of tumors of higher stage and grade than do non-smokers. The correlation between cigarette smoking and cancer is reportedly higher for bladder cancer than for lung cancer.

The prevalence of cigar smoking in patients with bladder cancer has not been well defined.

Occupational risks. The strongest association between work and bladder cancer is among aniline dye workers exposed to aromatic amines, with a relatively increased risk of 1.7–8.8. Other occupations with increased risk of urinary bladder cancer (UBC) due to exposure to carcinogens in the workplace are listed in Table 1.2.

TABLE 1.1

Known bladder carcinogens

- 2-Naphthylamine
- Benzidine
- 4-Aminobiphenyl
- Dichlorobenzidine
- Orthodianisidine

- Orthotolidine
- Phenacetin
- Chlornaphazine
- Cyclophosphamide

TABLE 1.2

Industries in which workers may be exposed to carcinogens

- Dye manufacture
- Rubber manufacture (especially tires and cables)
- Production of coal gas
- Sewage work
- Firelighter manufacture
- Pest control
- Textile printing
- Hairdressing

Dietary factors. Caffeine has been implicated in bladder cancer, but the relationship has been hard to define because of the widespread use of caffeine, as well as its association with a variety of other known carcinogens, such as those arising from smoking. Artificial sweeteners have also been implicated, but the studies undertaken involved extremely high doses, and more recent research has failed to clarify this relationship. At present, the consensus is that neither caffeine nor artificial sweeteners used in normal doses cause bladder cancer.

Drugs. Certain drugs, such as cyclophosphamide and phenacetin, have been linked with bladder cancer. Phenacetin, which is especially associated with tumors of the renal pelvis, is not licensed for pharmaceutical use in the UK and has been withdrawn in the USA, but is still used topically in hair-care products. Cyclophosphamide, too, has been linked with bladder cancer in both animal and human studies. The proportion of muscle-invasive tumors in patients is high, and the time between exposure and diagnosis is relatively short (6–13 years). Prophylactic administration of 2-mercaptoethanesulfonic acid (mesna) reduces the rate of cyclophosphamide-related cystitis and has even been suggested to reduce the risk of subsequent bladder cancer.

Radiation. Radiotherapy for cervical cancer is linked with a fourfold increase in the risk of bladder cancer.

Chronic infection or inflammation due to indwelling suprapubic catheters in patients with spinal cord injury has been linked to an increased incidence of bladder cancer, especially squamous cell cancer. A similar association has been noted in patients practicing intermittent self-catheterization in the presence of chronic urinary tract infection (UTI). Schistosomiasis, caused by the organism *Schistosoma haematobium* (Figure 1.1), is associated with an incidence of bladder cancer as high as 70% in areas of Egypt, where it is the most common cause of bladder cancer. While most such tumors are squamous cell cancers, transitional cell carcinomas are also found in association with schistosomiasis.

Fluid intake. The incidence of bladder cancer varies with level of fluid intake: the higher the intake, the lower the frequency of bladder cancer.

Chromosomal and genetic changes. Loss of heterozygosity of chromosome 9 (implying the presence of a specific gene located on that chromosome) seems to be associated with the genesis of low-grade superficial bladder cancer. In contrast, loss of heterozygosity

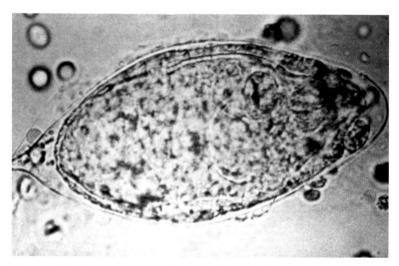

Figure 1.1 *Schistosoma haematobium*: infection with this parasite is endemic in parts of Africa and may cause squamous cell carcinoma of the bladder.

of chromosome 17, and specifically a mutation of the p53 suppressor gene, is associated with the development of carcinoma in situ (CIS), invasive and metastatic disease. More recently, mutations of the *Rb* (retinoblastoma) gene, and of p16 and p21, have been found to be linked to bladder cancer and its natural history. It is also relevant that the *RAS* gene was first identified in a cell line of bladder cancer.

Key points – epidemiology and etiology

- Bladder cancer is a common tumor and has a 3:1 male-to-female ratio.
- Each year approximately 10 000 people in the USA and 5 000 in the UK will die from bladder cancer.
- The commonest cause of bladder cancer is cigarette smoking.
- The genetic nature of an individual tumor determines its future behavior.

Key references

Bostwick DG. Natural history of early bladder cancer. *J Cell Biol* 1992;161(suppl):31–8.

Dalbagni G, Presti J, Reuter V et al. Genetic alterations in bladder cancer. *Lancet* 1993;342:469–71.

Michaud DS, Spiegelman D, Clinton SK et al. Fluid intake and the risk of bladder cancer in men. *N Engl J Med* 1999;340:1390–7.

Morrison AS, Buring JE, Verhoek WG et al. An international study of smoking and bladder cancer. *J Urol* 1984;131:650–4.

Parker SL, Tong T, Bolden S, Wingo PA. Cancer statistics, 1997. *CA Cancer J Clin* 1997;47:5–27.

Pattison S, Choong S, Corbishley CM, Bailey MJ. Squamous cell carcinoma of the bladder, intermittent self-catheterisation and urinary tract infection – is there an association? *BJU Int* 2001;88:441.

Thompson IM, Peek M, Rodriguez FR. The impact of cigarette smoking on stage, grade and number of recurrences in transitional cell carcinoma of the bladder. *J Urol* 1987;137:401–3.

Vineis P. The use of biomarkers in epidemiology: the example of bladder cancer. *Toxicol Lett* 1992;463:64–5.

Wolf H, Melsen F, Pedersen SE, Nielsen KT. Natural history of carcinoma in situ of the urinary bladder. *Scand J Urol Nephrol* 1994;157(suppl):147–51.

Histology

The following histological types of carcinoma occur in the bladder:
- transitional cell cancer (TCC)
  - papillary and superficial
  - solid and invasive
  - carcinoma in situ (CIS, also known as Tis)
- squamous cell carcinoma
- adenocarcinoma
- small-cell anaplastic bladder cancer
- bladder sarcoma
- choriocarcinoma.

In addition, field changes may be observed.

Transitional cell cancer (TCC). Derived from the transitional epithelium, TCC accounts for almost 90% of the bladder cancers seen in industrialized countries such as the USA and the UK (Figure 2.1). Most of the discussion on bladder cancer revolves around this type. Such tumors may be papillary and superficial (70–75%) or solid and invasive (20–25%). CIS is an additional and important type seen in about 10% of cases (sometimes as secondary CIS alongside another tumor). CIS is a flat, intraepithelial, anaplastic carcinoma, often with increased numbers of mitotic structures. In approximately half of all cases, CIS occurs as an isolated lesion (primary CIS), while in the remainder it occurs in association with either papillary or solid tumors (secondary CIS). When CIS and superficial bladder cancer coexist, the prognosis is worse than for superficial disease alone.

It should also be noted that TCC can coexist with elements of squamous and glandular differentiation. The classification of the tumor depends on the dominant histological type. In an important development in research, a common stem cell of origin has been identified in xenograft and cell culture studies. This stem cell type

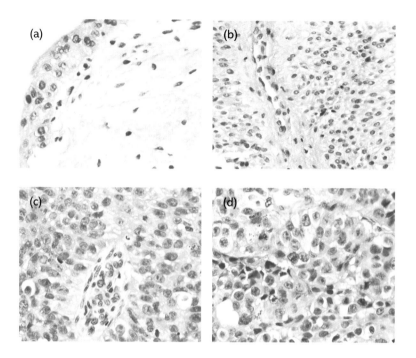

Figure 2.1 Histological sections through the urothelium. (a) Normal urothelium is 3–7 cells thick, and lies between a basement membrane and an intact layer of umbrella cells on the luminal surface. (b) In grade 1 papillary transitional cell carcinoma (TCC), urothelial cells have a slightly increased nucleus-to-cell ratio, and umbrella cells are lost. A fibrovascular stalk is usually prominent. (c) Grade 2 papillary TCC is associated with a large nucleus-to-cell ratio. There are occasional nucleoli, with some maintenance of cell polarity. (d) With grade 3 TCC, a wide range of cell shapes and sizes is seen. The nucleus-to-cell ratio is very high, mitosis is occasional to frequent, and many cells have multiple nucleoli.

has features of TCC as well as showing squamous and glandular differentiation within individual tumor cells. This may explain the phenomenon of non-TCC metastases (such as squamous cell carcinoma or adenocarcinoma) occurring in patients with pure TCC primary tumors.

Squamous cell carcinoma. Usually an invasive lesion, squamous cell carcinoma has a nodular, infiltrative growth pattern. It accounts for about 5–10% of bladder cancers in the USA and UK, but up to 70% of bladder cancers in areas where schistosomiasis is endemic, such as Egypt. It is also associated with chronic infection or inflammation, such as that due to indwelling suprapubic catheters.

Adenocarcinoma is a rare type of bladder carcinoma, making up about 2% of bladder cancers. Approximately 30–35% of adenocarcinomas are urachal in origin and location, while the remainder are associated with bladder exstrophy or are non-urachal in origin. The urachus is the remnant of the embryonic cavity, the allantois; it usually forms a fibrous cord connecting the bladder to the umbilicus.

Adenocarcinomas are usually solitary, high grade and ulcerative. They are indistinguishable histologically from adenocarcinoma of the colon or rectum, and clinical determination of the source is often difficult. Many patients have a poor prognosis because the tumor is already at an advanced stage at the time of diagnosis. Urachal adenocarcinomas in particular tend to be asymptomatic until late in the course of the disease, since they arise in a minimally functional portion of the bladder.

Uncommon variants have also been identified. Most prominent of these is small-cell anaplastic bladder cancer, which is similar to the more common small-cell cancer of the lung. This histological pattern is associated with rapid growth and early metastasis. The cells have a high nucleus-to-cytoplasm ratio, and grow in sheets or nests of cells. This variant should be distinguished from undifferentiated uroepithelial carcinoma, which is the least differentiated of the TCCs. Less commonly, small-cell anaplastic bladder cancer is squamous or glandular in origin.

Very rarely, bladder sarcomas are detected, usually on histological review of a cystectomy specimen.

Perhaps the least common variant of bladder cancer is choriocarcinoma, which is usually associated with the production of human chorionic gonadotropin, and which has been most often reported in Far East Asian populations.

'Field changes' of a probable premalignant nature are often found in association with bladder cancer, and range from atypia to mild or severe dysplasia. The recognition of such changes is important in determining the future risk of recurrence or progression. Normal transitional epithelium has a superficial layer of large, flat umbrella cells, beneath which are between three and seven layers of regular cells. These lie above a basement membrane that separates the mucosa from the underlying muscularis. The WHO has recently reclassified urothelial neoplasms and recognizes hyperplasia as well as four types of atypia. These include dysplasia (low-grade intraurothelial neoplasia) and CIS (high-grade intraurothelial neoplasia, formerly classified as severe dysplasia). Atypia indicates that an increased number of cell layers is present, with loss of polarity of a still intact umbrella layer. Dysplasia refers to an increase in the size of nuclei that are basally located and exhibit loss of the usual polarity. The cell layers are not increased in number.

Staging

Tumor–nodes–metastases (TNM) staging is the system most widely used in the management of bladder cancer (Figure 2.2). Accurate staging and grading of UBC is essential, as it determines the most effective treatment. Understaging and undergrading may result in use of inadequate adjuvant therapy or incorrect selection of primary management options (see Chapters 6 and 7, pages 41 and 53) and, thus, in tumor progression.

In the most recent edition of the *Staging Manual of the American Joint Committee on Cancer*, mention is made of the prognostic significance of mutation of p53 and other genes. Molecular prognostication may assume a greater role in clinical management in the near future. For example, there are data to suggest that p53 mutation is associated, stage for stage, with a worse prognosis (e.g. pT2 tumors with p53 mutation have a lower survival than pT2 tumors with wild-type p53).

The phenomenon of stage migration has become important in the assessment of the clinical stage of bladder cancer. Increasing precision in non-invasive staging has resulted in the ability to detect

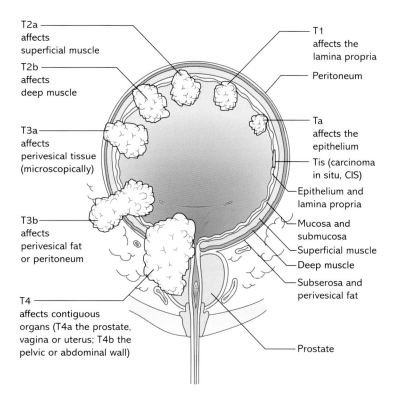

T2a affects superficial muscle

T2b affects deep muscle

T3a affects perivesical tissue (microscopically)

T3b affects perivesical fat or peritoneum

T4 affects contiguous organs (T4a the prostate, vagina or uterus; T4b the pelvic or abdominal wall)

T1 affects the lamina propria

Peritoneum

Ta affects the epithelium

Tis (carcinoma in situ, CIS)

Epithelium and lamina propria

Mucosa and submucosa

Superficial muscle

Deep muscle

Subserosa and perivesical fat

Prostate

Figure 2.2 TNM staging of bladder cancer, based on the level of invasion into or through the bladder wall, the involvement of lymph nodes and distant sites of disease.

smaller amounts of invasive and metastatic disease. Current staging modalities are able to detect lymph-node deposits and liver or lung metastases, for example, at a much earlier stage of development than was the case 20 years ago. As a result, patients with less extensive disease are being included in management programs for invasive or metastatic disease, and it is thus likely that results will appear to improve, based solely on the classification of patients in each category of invasive or metastatic disease. Likewise, in the 1970s, patients were treated with curative intent for invasive bladder cancer when imaging failed to detect significant para-aortic lymphadenopathy; such cases would now be treated as metastatic, and are thus removed from the denominator of surgical or radiation cases. One must bear this change in mind when interpreting the literature and assessing the extent of progress in the past 20 years.

Grading

A system of three grades for evaluating anaplasia – 1, 2 and 3 for well, moderately and poorly differentiated, respectively – has been adopted by most pathologists (Table 2.1).

Patterns of recurrence and spread

Most superficial Ta and T1 tumors can be completely resected endoscopically and treated successfully without cystectomy. Approximately 40% of patients with such tumors will have no recurrence after resection of the primary tumor, but initially this subgroup of patients cannot be distinguished with certainty from those whose tumors will recur (stratification criteria are given in Chapter 6). Of those patients who do experience recurrence, 20–30% may suffer progression to a higher stage (see Chapter 6). Consequently, vigilant surveillance is necessary, as is judicious use of intravesical agents to decrease the likelihood of recurrence and progression in high-risk patients (for example, those with large or multiple tumors, high-grade lesions, or superficial tumors with associated CIS or severe dysplasia).

Most recurrences are found in the bladder, although 4–10% of patients develop a tumor in the upper tract and a similar number may develop a tumor in the prostatic urethra. Conversely, 40% of

TABLE 2.1

Grading system for anaplasia in bladder cancer

Grade 1:	Tumors have the least degree of anaplasia compatible with the diagnosis of cancer
Grade 2:	Tumors have a degree of anaplasia between grades 1 and 3
Grade 3:	Tumors have the most severe degree of anaplasia

patients who have an initial TCC of the renal pelvis will subsequently develop transitional cell tumors in the bladder.

CIS has a high rate of progression to muscle-invasive disease if it is not eradicated with adjuvant therapy or surgical resection. It may also spread to lymph nodes without first going through a recognized progression to muscle-invasive disease.

Muscle-invasive disease has a high rate of direct spread to regional structures such as pelvic muscles, lymphatic spread to regional lymph nodes, and hematogenous spread to lungs, viscera and bones.

Mortality

Mortality due to TCC is directly related to the pathological stage and grade of bladder cancer. For those with Ta and low-grade T1 tumors, 5-year disease-specific survival should exceed 95%. For patients with high-grade T1 cancers or CIS, reported 5-year survival without adjuvant therapy may be as low as 50%. If adequate bacillus Calmette–Guérin (BCG) immunotherapy is used, 5-year survival should approach 80–85%. Patients with T2/T3aN0M0 disease have only a 60–70% 5-year survival, despite complete surgical excision. This surprisingly low disease-specific survival is due to the progression of subclinical 'micrometastases', which were present at the time of cystectomy but were not radiologically detectable. Some 80% of these cases develop within 2 years of cystectomy, with the remainder presenting in the 2 years thereafter.

Patients with T4 TCC have a 5-year survival of only 10–20%; the survival of those with T4a disease is at the upper end of this range. Individuals with para-aortic or distant lymph-node metastases but no visceral disease are occasionally cured by chemotherapy, but the 5-year survival lies in the range of 20–40%. Patients with visceral metastases have a 5-year survival, irrespective of chemotherapy, of only around 10%. Independent adverse prognostic determinants for patients with metastatic disease include poor performance status, weight loss and elevated liver function test results and alkaline phosphatase levels. Interestingly, sex and age are not independent prognostic variables.

Patients with adenocarcinoma or squamous carcinoma have a 5-year survival of more than 50% following complete surgical excision, provided that the lymph nodes are clear. However, if metastases are present, the prognosis is grim (see Chemotherapy in Chapters 7 and 8). Patients with small-cell anaplastic carcinoma or choriocarcinoma are rarely cured, as these tumors are usually associated with extensive disease at presentation. The prognosis for bladder sarcomas is determined by histological subtype, extent of disease and performance status.

Key points – pathology

- Low-grade superficial bladder tumors may recur, but progress to muscle invasion in less than 5% of cases.
- High-grade superficial bladder cancer will progress if not adequately treated with resection and bacillus Calmette–Guérin.
- Carcinoma in situ, whether primary or secondary, is a high-risk tumor.
- Muscle-invasive disease requires radical treatment with either cystectomy or radiotherapy.
- Up to 30% of patients with high-grade superficial tumors and up to 70% with muscle-invasive disease may die of bladder cancer.
- Metastatic disease has a poor prognosis, particularly if hepatic or bone metastases are present.

Key references

Green FL, Page DL, Fleming ID et al., eds. *American Joint Committee on Cancer Cancer Staging Manual,* 6th edn. Berlin: Springer, 2002.

Presti JC Jr, Reuter VE, Galan T et al. Molecular genetic alterations in superficial and locally advanced human bladder cancer. *Cancer Res* 1991;51:5405–9.

Raghavan D. Molecular targeting and pharmacogenomics in the management of advanced bladder cancer. *Cancer* 2003:97(8 suppl); 2083–9.

Sandberg AA, Berger CS. Review of chromosome studies urological tumors. II. Cytogenetics and molecular genetics of bladder cancer. *J Urol* 1994;151:545–60.

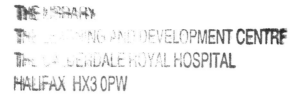

The classic presenting symptom of a patient with a bladder tumor is painless hematuria. This symptom is usually taken seriously by the patient and the primary care physician, and appropriate action initiated. However, other presentations are not uncommon (Table 3.1) and are sometimes unrecognized as an indication of serious underlying pathology.

TABLE 3.1

Presenting symptoms

Symptom	Description
Painless hematuria	Visible passage of blood in urine, without associated pain, frequency or dysuria. Up to 30% of patients with painless hematuria will have urinary tract malignancy
Microscopic hematuria	Presence of red blood cells in the urine of insufficient quantity to be visible to the naked eye, without urologic symptoms. About 4–6% of these patients will have malignant disease of the urinary tract
Irritative symptoms	Dysuria, frequency, suprapubic pain with a full bladder. Some 25% of patients with bladder tumors will have one or more of these symptoms
Recurrent urinary tract infection	In older (50+ years) patients with recurrent bacterial cystitis, the possibility of an underlying tumor should be considered
Symptoms of local or distant spread	Loin pain, weight loss, malaise, anorexia, bone pain, pathological fracture, cough, headache, abdominal pain

Painless hematuria

Painless hematuria may occur at the beginning, at the end or throughout the stream of urine. It may be profuse, so that the patient complains of passing pure blood, and the urine may contain clots, or there may be only a slight pink discoloration of the urine. If there have been clots in the bladder for some time, they may impart a rusty color to the urine. Any patient complaining of these symptoms should be referred to a urologist immediately. Patients will sometimes ignore a single episode of bleeding and delay seeking advice until the bleeding recurs. The resulting delay in diagnosis and treatment may make treatment more difficult and reduce the chance of cure.

Hematuria, either painless or microscopic, is the sole presenting symptom in 60–80% of patients with carcinoma of the bladder. However, up to 20% of patients with bladder cancer will not have hematuria at the time of presentation.

Asymptomatic microscopic hematuria

As screening programs and medical examinations for insurance purposes become more widespread, the finding of microscopic or dipstick hematuria is increasing. Because this is now such a common finding, the topic of microscopic hematuria is covered separately in Chapter 5. Microscopic hematuria may be part of the spectrum of painless hematuria, but its sensitivity and specificity are low for detection of bladder cancer.

Irritative symptoms

Dysuria, increased frequency and urgency are usually due to UTI. Because irritative symptoms are common and are usually not associated with serious disease, it is easy for patients and their primary care physicians to dismiss them. However, if infection is absent or symptoms persist after the infection has been treated, the possibility of an underlying bladder carcinoma must be considered and the patient should be referred to a urologist.

Irritative symptoms are especially common in patients with CIS. Suprapubic pain when the bladder is full can also be caused by carcinoma of the bladder.

Urinalysis in patients with irritative symptoms due to CIS or invasive cancer will usually reveal red or white blood cells, and if urine cytology is requested, it may detect malignant cells.

Recurrent urinary traction infections

Recurrent infections are sometimes due to the presence of a bladder tumor. A single infection in a man, or two or more infections in a woman, should be investigated. The likelihood of a malignant etiology in patients under 50 years of age is, however, very small.

Symptoms of local or distant spread

Patients sometimes present with systemic symptoms due to advanced carcinoma of the bladder. Loin pain can be caused by ureteric obstruction by an invasive bladder tumor (Figure 3.1). The pain is usually a dull ache in the renal angle, and may or may not coincide with other symptoms such as hematuria. Occasionally, infection occurs in an obstructed system, giving rise to severe symptoms of pyelonephritis.

Coughing, dyspnea or chest pain may be due to pulmonary metastases (Figure 3.2); the cough is usually non-productive. Pleuritic chest pain may also be present.

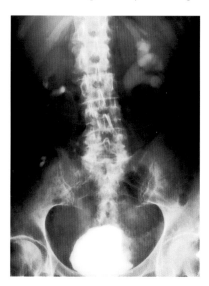

Figure 3.1 Intravenous urogram showing ureteric obstruction by a bladder tumor. Obstruction is usually a sign of an invasive tumor.

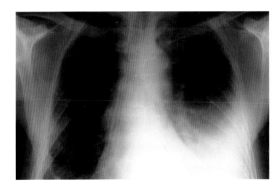

Figure 3.2 Chest radiograph showing multiple pulmonary metastases.

Anorexia, nausea, weight loss and malaise may result from renal failure caused by bilateral ureteric obstruction, or from the systemic effects of the tumor itself. Bone pain or pathological fractures may result from skeletal metastases (Figure 3.3); the pain is unrelieved by rest and can be very severe. Anemia and hypercalcemia may occur as metabolic complications of advanced disease; leukocytosis is occasionally associated with the elaboration of colony-stimulating factors by the tumor.

Although uncommon as a presenting feature, headache or disordered thought processes may indicate underlying brain metastases. These symptoms may be due to cerebral cortical deposits or carcinomatous meningitis.

Delay in diagnosis

Although it is difficult to prove that delay in diagnosis affects prognosis, a recent study goes some way to demonstrating a

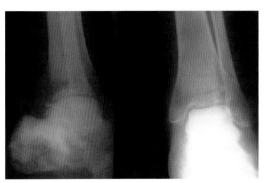

Figure 3.3 Bone destruction by secondary deposits from an invasive bladder tumor. When such deposits are present in a weight-bearing bone. pathological fracture may occur.

25

relationship. It therefore seems advisable to ensure prompt diagnosis and treatment for patients with bladder cancer. Delays may occur for a variety of reasons.

- Presentation by the patient may be delayed because of the patient's anxiety about the cause of the symptoms, fear of primary care physicians or hospitals or ignorance of the significance of symptoms.
- Referral by the primary care physician to a specialist may be delayed owing to ignorance of the significance of the symptoms or limited access to specialist healthcare (waiting times for clinic appointments).
- Diagnosis by the specialist may be delayed because of waiting times for investigations, waiting time to attend follow-up clinics for results or waiting lists for cystoscopy.

Taken together, these factors mean that the average time from the patient first noticing a symptom to the time of treatment of the bladder tumor varies in different studies from a few weeks to more than a year.

In an attempt to streamline the diagnosis and treatment of patients with symptoms suggestive of bladder cancer, many hospitals now offer a hematuria clinic at which patients can be seen within a week of referral. The service should be able to perform urine cytology and dipstick analysis for blood and leukocytes, intravenous urography or ultrasound and plain radiology of the urinary tract, and flexible cystoscopy, all on the same day. This allows a diagnosis to be made and treatment planned expeditiously.

Key points – clinical presentation

- Painless hematuria is the commonest presentation of urinary bladder cancer (UBC).
- A single episode of hematuria should prompt urgent referral to a urologist.
- Unexplained irritative symptoms may be due to UBC, especially to carcinoma in situ.
- Recurrent infections may indicate an underlying tumor.
- Delay in treatment adversely affects prognosis.
- Hematuria clinics allow rapid diagnosis and reduce time to treatment.

Key references

Hastie KJ, Hamdy FC, Collins MC, Williams JL. Upper tract tumours following cystectomy for bladder cancer. Is routine intravenous urography worthwhile? *Br J Urol* 1991;67:29–31.

Lynch TH, Waymont B, Dunn JA et al. Repeat testing for haematuria and underlying urological pathology. *Br J Urol* 1994;74:730–2.

Mommsen S, Aargard J, Sell A. Presenting symptoms, treatment delay and survival in bladder cancer. *Scand J Urol Nephrol* 1983;17: 163–7.

Wallace DM, Bryan RT, Dunn JA et al. Delay and survival in bladder cancer. *BJU Int* 2002;89:868–78.

4 Investigations

History
A thorough history should be obtained from all patients presenting with symptoms suggestive of bladder cancer. The history should cover smoking, possible carcinogen exposure in the workplace, previous bladder tumor resection and any change in bowel habits or stool characteristics. Direct questioning may reveal hematuria for 6–12 months prior to presentation.

Examination
Physical examination is usually unremarkable in cases of superficial bladder cancer unless acute urinary retention is present with bladder distension. In men, a careful rectal examination should be carried out to exclude prostatic disease such as cancer or benign enlargement, both of which may cause many of the same symptoms as bladder cancer, and to rule out gross extension of bladder cancer. A careful pelvic examination in women is equally important. A thorough nodal examination should be undertaken, including supraclavicular lymph nodes, as well as assessment for hepatic or pulmonary involvement.

Detailed investigation
Urinalysis should begin with dipstick testing for the presence of red blood cells and, if the result is positive, microscopic analysis should be performed for confirmation. The presence of nitrates or leukocytes should prompt urine culture to look for infection.

Several recently developed tests for urinary markers of urothelial malignancy are commercially available, and tests for other urinary markers are still at the laboratory stage. At present, none of the tests alone is sufficiently sensitive to replace cystoscopy in diagnosing or excluding UBC. They may prove useful in dictating the frequency of cystoscopy for recurrence in patients with known bladder cancer. Table 4.1 shows the sensitivity and specificity of some of these markers.

Imaging. The upper tracts should be imaged in all patients with symptoms suggestive of bladder cancer. In the investigation of hematuria (the commonest presentation of bladder cancer), the imaging can be performed either by intravenous urography (IVU) or by ultrasound plus a plain radiograph of the kidneys, ureters and bladder (KUB). The diagnostic yield from these procedures is equivalent, but ultrasound is better at detecting solid renal masses than IVU, and IVU (Figure 4.1) is better at demonstrating upper-tract urothelial tumors. If one imaging modality yields negative results, and cystoscopy is also normal, the other type of imaging should be carried out.

TABLE 4.1

Sensitivity and specificity of tests for urinary markers of bladder cancer

Test	Sensitivity (%)	Specificity (%)	Comment
Cytology	49.8	96.6	Readily available
BTA stat	67.7	65.8	False positives with infection/hematuria
BTA TRAK	71.1	62.0	Complex test*
NMP22	64.3	71.2	Complex test*
Telomerase	74	89	Complex test,* not commercially available
HA/HAase	91	86	Complex test,* not commercially available
Immunocyst	68	79	Complex test*
F/FDP	68	86	No longer commercially available

* Requires reference laboratory.
BTA, bladder tumor antigen; F/FDP, fibrin/fibrinogen degradation products; HA/HAase, hyaluronic acid/hyaluronidase; NMP, nuclear matrix protein.

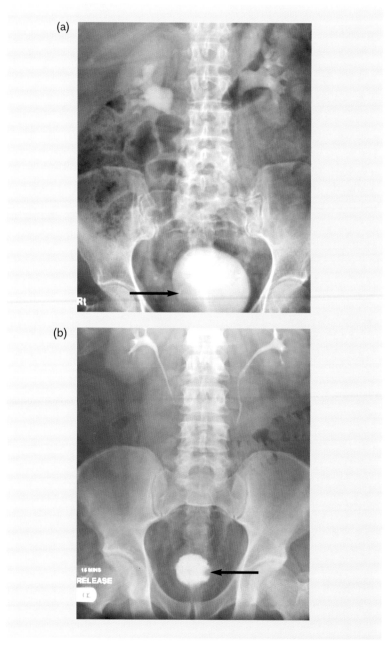

Figure 4.1 Intravenous urograms showing (a) a large bladder carcinoma,
(b) a small polyp.

Improvements in contrast technology have increased the accuracy and utility of CT scanning, and it has recently been suggested that this approach should be used as the primary imaging modality. However, in many countries, including the UK, limited access to CT scanners makes this impractical at present. In the USA, CT scanning is used routinely.

If a patient is found to have low-grade superficial bladder cancer on biopsy, no further imaging is required. High-risk superficial disease can be associated with occult lymph-node metastases, and computed tomography (CT) or magnetic resonance imaging (MRI) may be considered in these patients. However, if muscle-invasive disease is present, staging with chest, abdominal and pelvic CT scanning is necessary. This should identify visceral metastatic disease within the limits of resolution of the scanner. Pelvic MRI scanning may give more accurate details about local spread of invasive bladder cancer.

Bone scans are indicated in patients with invasive disease only when they have symptoms suggesting bone involvement (i.e. pain) or in the presence of elevated bone markers (alkaline phosphatase).

Cystoscopy is required to determine the presence or absence of small tumors that may not be seen in the bladder views of the IVU. It can usually be accomplished under local anesthetic with a flexible cystoscope (Figure 4.2). If a bladder tumor is obvious on the IVU, then cystoscopy under local anesthetic may be omitted. Instead, the

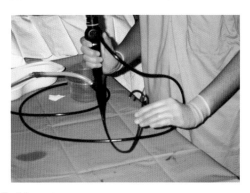

Figure 4.2 A flexible cystoscope.

patient may be taken directly to the operating suite for rigid endoscopy under general anesthesia, with simultaneous resection or biopsy of the tumor. Before and after tumor resection, with the patient under anesthesia, a careful bimanual examination should be performed to identify a mass in the bladder.

Cytological examination of exfoliated cells should be performed in cases of high-grade tumor after resection and after any hematuria has cleared. A bladder wash for cytology should also be obtained at the time of cystoscopy if areas that might be CIS or ulcers are seen instead of obvious tumor. Cytology may be helpful in following such patients for signs of recurrence, as well as ensuring that all disease present at initial diagnosis has been diagnosed and treated adequately. Cytology is relatively insensitive in low-grade disease and is therefore not warranted.

Expert pathological interpretation of both histology and cytology specimens is critical. Recent reports indicate a rate of discordance of at least 30% among pathologists, including many who specialize in uropathology. Because many treatment and prognostic decisions are based on fine distinctions between grade (3 versus 1 or 2), invasion (T1 versus T2) and field changes (CIS versus mild or moderate dysplasia), it is important that both understaging and overstaging of bladder cancers be minimized. Second-opinion pathology should be routine if the initial reporting pathologist sees only an occasional case of bladder cancer.

Transurethral resection of the tumor(s) is the mainstay of both diagnosis and initial management. If limited papillary disease is present, as is most often the case, no additional therapy may be required other than regular cystoscopic surveillance. Complete resection may be possible if the tumor is small, solid and muscle-invasive only (Figure 4.3). However, extensive resections of large, invasive tumors may serve no useful purpose, because cystectomy may be needed shortly. In addition, the risk of postoperative bleeding and clot retention is increased. Deep biopsy at the juncture of the tumor and the muscular wall may be sufficient to confirm the diagnosis of muscle involvement.

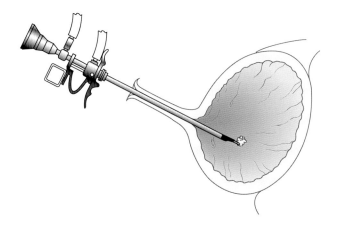

Figure 4.3 Transurethral resection of a small, solid, muscle-invasive tumor.

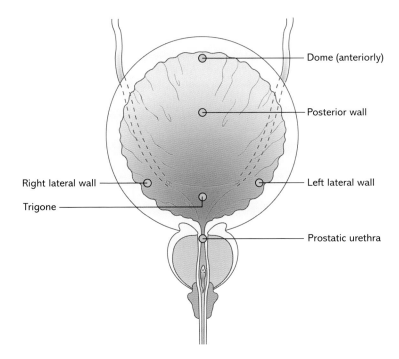

Dome (anteriorly)

Posterior wall

Right lateral wall

Trigone

Left lateral wall

Prostatic urethra

Figure 4.4 Sites for directed mucosal biopsies of the bladder.

Biopsy. Mucosal biopsies should be performed in selected cases to rule out or diagnose associated field changes (Figure 4.4). Small, obviously low-grade papillary and superficial tumors do not warrant such biopsies.

Biopsies should be performed under the following circumstances:
- cases of multiple papillary tumors
- tumors that appear more solid but are resectable
- bladders with erythematous areas that may represent CIS
- if chemoradiation with bladder conservation is being considered
- to determine whether the prostate/bladder neck region is free of CIS in patients for whom orthotopic bladder reconstruction is planned after cystectomy.

Biopsies might also be obtained circumferentially around small, solid, apparently invasive tumors away from the bladder base or bladder neck in selected cases where partial cystectomy might be considered for definitive therapy.

Key points – investigations

- The investigation of a patient with suspected bladder cancer should include urinalysis, upper-tract imaging and cystoscopy.
- Expert pathological review of biopsy specimens is critical to determining appropriate treatment.
- Cross-sectional imaging (CT or MRI) is used to stage invasive disease.
- Urinary markers are not yet sufficiently sensitive for diagnosis, but may be useful in following up patients with superficial disease.

Key references

Bailey MJ. Urinary markers in bladder cancer. *BJU Int* 2003;91: 772–3.

Mufti GR, Singh M. Value of random mucosal biopsies in the management of superficial bladder cancer. *Eur Urol* 1992;22:288–93.

Palou J, Farina LA, Villavicencio H, Vicente J. Upper tract urothelial tumor after transurethral resection for bladder tumor. *Eur Urol* 1992; 21:110–14.

Tosoni I, Wagner U, Sauter G et al. Clinical significance of interobserver differences in the staging and grading of superficial bladder cancer. *BJU Int* 2000;85:48–53.

Witjes JA, Kiemeney LALM, Verbeek ALM et al.; Dutch South East Cooperative Urological Group. Random bladder biopsies and the risk of recurrent superficial bladder cancer. A prospective study in 1026 patients. *World J Urol* 1992;10: 231–4.

Asymptomatic microscopic hematuria may be caused by any of the conditions causing frank painless hematuria, and should be appropriately investigated.

Recently, the value of testing for microscopic hematuria has been called into question, but it is still standard practice in the UK and the USA to investigate any patient found to test positive.

Excretion of red blood cells

Excretion of red blood cells (RBCs) at a rate of 0–1 million per 24 hours is considered normal. If urine is centrifuged and the deposit examined using a high-power microscope, this number of red cells would equate to 0–5 RBCs per high-power field (HPF). Thus, the finding of red cells in numbers greater than this may be considered abnormal. It has been suggested that a finding of 5 RBCs/HPF should represent the threshold for instigating investigation in asymptomatic individuals. However, because there is little uniformity among laboratories in the method of preparing urine samples for microscopy, the question of what constitutes a normal number of RBCs in urine is difficult to answer definitely.

Collection of urine samples

In order to avoid unnecessary investigation, it is important to collect urine samples in a way that will avoid contamination.

- Withdraw the foreskin and clean the glans.
- Do not take samples when the individual is menstruating.
- Do not take samples after vigorous exercise.
- Always use freshly voided samples – bacterial breakdown of urinary constituents could yield false positives on dipstick testing and false-positive cultures for infection.

False-negative reactions occur with high vitamin C levels or if there is contamination with formalin.

Reagent testing

Dipsticks are widely used as an economical and simple screening test for the presence of blood, hemoglobin, protein, nitrites, glucose and leukocytes in urine samples (Figure 5.1). The reaction used to detect RBCs or hemoglobin is peroxidase-based, and commercial reagent strips are sufficiently sensitive to detect 2–5 RBCs/HPF. As dipsticks may be so sensitive to blood in the urine that they yield a positive result at a lower threshold than that at which further investigation is warranted (i.e. 5 RBCs/HPF), weak positive dipstick results for hematuria should be confirmed by microscopic urinalysis with the threshold for evaluation set at 5 RBCs/HPF. This procedure will decrease the number of investigations following false-positive dipstick results. However, as hematuria can be intermittent, a 2 or 3+ reaction in an appropriately collected specimen of urine should prompt investigation even if results from subsequent urine microscopy are negative.

Hematuria, whether macroscopic or microscopic, can be intermittent even when there is a urologic malignancy, so repeat testing to confirm the finding is not helpful in defining a high-risk group.

Age must be taken into account when assessing microscopic hematuria. In all reported studies, the number of patients under

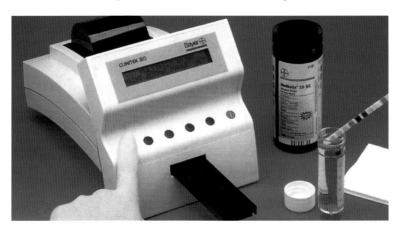

Figure 5.1 A reagent strip and equipment to test for blood and other substances in the urine.

40 years of age who were found to have a serious urologic cause for their hematuria was very small. Patients in this age group with hematuria and proteinuria should initially be referred to a nephrologist. As bladder cancer or renal carcinoma may occasionally occur in patients under 40 years of age, subsequent urologic investigation may be indicated if the nephrologist finds no explanation for the hematuria. Anyone over 40 years of age with hematuria detected by a dipstick test (if the test has been correctly performed and false positives excluded) should be investigated by a urologist. Some 2–5% of patients over 40 years of age with a positive dipstick test result will be found to have a bladder tumor, another 5–10% will have significant pathology such as stone disease, prostate cancer or renal cancer, and the majority will have no detectable cause. In those in whom no abnormality is detected, there is no increased risk of developing urologic disease in the future.

Diagnostic workup

Patients with asymptomatic microscopic hematuria (AMH) should have a full workup, as for frank hematuria. Ultrasound of the renal tract together with a standard radiograph can be substituted for an IVU, but a small TCC of the upper tract may be missed. Therefore, if negative results are found with one imaging option, the other should be requested.

If proteinuria is found in association with hematuria, a nephrological cause should be sought. Phase-contrast microscopy of the urine may identify dysmorphic or crenellated RBCs characteristic of renal disease. The results of investigations in patients with hematuria are shown in Table 5.1. Other, population-based, studies on the use of microscopic hematuria in diagnosis have shown that 2–22% of those with microscopic hematuria have bladder cancer. In one such study of 2700 subjects aged 35–55 years, 13% had one or more RBCs/HPF detected in a spun deposit of urine, but only 2% of this group had serious urologic disease. It is difficult to account for this wide variation in results, but patient selection and techniques of urine collection

TABLE 5.1

Results of investigations in 395 patients with one or more episodes of hematuria

Diagnosis	Patients			Total (%)
	MH	ASM	SM	
No urologic abnormality	60	52	44	156 (39)
Urinary tract infection	45	5	39	89 (22)
Benign prostatic hyperplasia	44	7	6	57 (14)
Bladder tumor	26	3	2	31 (8)
Stone disease	10	8	2	20 (5)
Renal carcinoma	6	0	0	6 (1.5)
Carcinoma of the prostate	2	3	1	6 (1.5)
Urethral stricture	2	2	1	5 (1.3)
Other (benign)	18	4	2	24 (6)

ASM, asymptomatic microscopic hematuria; MH, macroscopic hematuria;
SM, symptomatic microscopic hematuria.
Data from Lynch et al. 1994.

and analysis may partly explain the differences, as may varying incidence in the subject group. The vast majority of studies have suggested an incidence of bladder cancer in AMH of no more than 5%.

Significance of a negative diagnostic workup

Follow-up studies have been undertaken to quantify the risk of missing a lesion on the standard workup for hematuria. For example, in a study involving 155 patients, no significant pathology was found over a 20-year period. There is therefore no need to retest patients who have been thoroughly evaluated and yielded only negative results. It must be stressed that this does not mean the individual concerned can ignore symptoms of urinary tract disease in the future – new pathology can of course develop, and macroscopic hematuria would require re-investigation.

Key points – microscopic hematuria

- Attention to the means of collection of the urine sample and the freshness of the reagent strips will minimize false-positive dipstick test results.
- Asymptomatic microscopic hematuria (AMH), whether on dipstick test or on microscopy, should be investigated as for macroscopic hematuria.
- The diagnostic yield for investigating AMH is lower than for macroscopic hematuria.
- In patients under 40 years of age, nephrological causes for AMH should be sought.
- If the diagnostic workup is negative, further testing is unnecessary.

Key references

Addis T. The number of formed elements in the urinary sediment of normal individuals. *J Clin Invest* 1926;2:409–15.

Frennis S, Heedrick G, Holt C et al. Centrifugation techniques and reagent strips in the assessment of microhaematuria. *J Clin Pathol* 1977;30:336–40.

Lynch TH, Waymont B, Dunn JA et al. Repeat testing for haematuria and underlying urological pathology. *Br J Urol* 1994;74:730–2.

Malmström PU. Time to abandon testing for microscopic haematuria in adults? *BMJ* 2003;326:813–15.

Sells H, Cox R. Undiagnosed haematuria revisited: a follow-up of 146 patients. *BJU Int* 2001;88:6–8.

Yasuma T, Koikawa Y, Uozumi J et al. Clinical study of asymptomatic microscopic haematuria. *Int J Urol Nephrol* 1994;26:1–6.

Basic principles

The UK National Institute for Health and Clinical Excellence has published a manual for *Improving Outcomes in Urological Cancers*. Key points in the manual's recommendations on the management of urologic cancers are listed below.

- All new tumors should be discussed by a multidisciplinary team (MDT).
- The management of high-risk superficial cancer should be discussed by the specialist MDT.
- Cystectomies should be carried out at a center where at least 50 radical prostatectomies and cystectomies are performed each year.
- Patients should be fully involved in choosing their treatment.

Prognostic factors

Following transurethral resection of the initial tumor and directed biopsies of mucosa with abnormal appearance, patients with non-invasive, superficial tumors (Ta or T1) may be stratified according to a number of prognostic factors. Table 6.1 shows the grouping of those factors into favorable and unfavorable initial tumor characteristics.

Histological grade and stage are the most useful prognostic factors to date. Without adjuvant therapy after surgery, recurrent tumors will be seen in no more than 50% of patients with grade 1 tumors, but in 80% of those with grade 3 tumors. Progression to muscle-invasive disease is rare for grade 1 tumors, but is seen in 11% of grade 2 tumors and in 50–80% of grade 3 tumors, depending on histological classification, extent of resected biopsy material and a series of other prognostic factors discussed below. Similarly, an initial Ta tumor progresses to grade T2 or higher in only 4% of patients, while such progression is seen in 30% of patients with T1

41

TABLE 6.1

Practical classification of superficial bladder cancers

By superficial tumor characteristics

Favorable	Unfavorable
Single tumor	Multiple tumors
Stage Ta	Stage T1
Low grade	High grade
No field changes	Carcinoma in situ
Diploid	Aneuploid
Negative cytology	Positive cytology

By characteristics and history of recurrence

Nuisance	Troublesome	Dangerous
Favorable characteristics, single occurrence or infrequent recurrences	Favorable characteristics but frequent recurrences	Unfavorable characteristics present at any occurrence or recurrence

tumors, 50% of those with CIS, and up to 80% of those with T1 tumors associated with CIS.

Single versus multiple tumors. The next strongest indicator of prognosis is the number of tumors. Over 60% of patients with three or more tumors at initial presentation will develop recurrent tumors, compared with 30–40% of those who have only one or two tumors at initial presentation.

Atypia, dysplasia and CIS. Mucosal or field changes of atypia, dysplasia and CIS found on random or directed biopsies are ominous indicators of outcome. Progression to muscle invasion is seen in only 7% of those who have a papillary tumor associated with normal mucosa, but in 36% if atypia is present, and in up to 80% if CIS is present.

Prognostic groups

Patients can be stratified into low-, intermediate- and high-risk groups; future therapy, as well as surveillance, may be tailored accordingly.

Low-risk, 'nuisance' tumors. Patients with a solitary, low-grade Ta lesion are at low risk of recurrence or progression. No adjuvant therapy need be given, as the cost and inconvenience of such therapy cannot be justified. Furthermore, recent experience suggests that if the first surveillance cystoscopy is negative, the interval before the following cystoscopy can be extended to 9 months, and thereafter they may be performed annually. Patients who do develop a recurrence of similar stage and grade have been shown to benefit from intravesical chemotherapy.

Intermediate-risk tumors. Patients with multiple, low-grade Ta tumors are at intermediate risk of recurrence or progression, particularly if atypia or dysplasia is also present. Similarly, patients with frequent recurrences of low-grade Ta tumors require surgical resection for each recurrence; this interferes with the patient's life and usually requires medical intervention (including repeated cystoscopies), although not usually threatening to life or bladder preservation. These patients should initially receive a course of intravesical therapy following resection (see below). In Europe, the usual treatment is intravesical cytotoxic chemotherapy, but in the USA, BCG is usually used.

High-risk tumors. Patients who present with CIS and/or high-grade papillary tumors have a risk of recurrence of 80% and progression rates of 40–70%. Whenever the pathology report of a resected tumor shows T1G3 disease and/or CIS, intravesical therapy with BCG should be used as an adjuvant. Recurrence or persistence of disease after one course of BCG places the patient at a greater likelihood of progression, but approximately one-third of such patients nevertheless respond to a second course. Thus, while most authorities would recommend cystectomy for non-responders to the first course of BCG, some urologists consider it reasonable to delay cystectomy for a second course of therapy. However, care should be taken not to delay cystectomy until after the tumor has invaded or metastasized.

Intravesical therapy

Anticancer drugs have been used intravesically (Figure 6.1) for bladder cancer for approximately 30 years, with most data demonstrating a modest beneficial effect in prevention of recurrence but not in prevention of progression in stage. Commonly used agents with demonstrated activity include thiotepa, doxorubicin, epirubicin and mitomycin C. Doxorubicin and mitomycin C are the preferred agents because their high molecular mass reduces systemic absorption. Thiotepa is a potential carcinogen, and its low molecular mass makes absorption through a denuded urothelium a possible hazard.

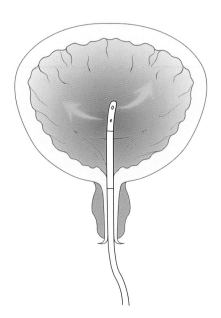

Figure 6.1 Intravesical therapy. The chemo-therapeutic agent is instilled into the bladder with a disposable catheter under urethral anesthesia. The patient is asked to retain the solution for a minimum of an hour, and then expel it by voiding normally. The surgeon may also ask the patient to move around, thus causing fluid shifts within the bladder cavity, in order to coat the lining of the bladder with the cytotoxic solution.

Chemotherapy. Intravesical chemotherapy has three uses:
- prophylactic
- therapeutic
- adjunctive.

Chemotherapeutic drugs have demonstrated limited therapeutic value in eradicating existing disease, such as residual tumors or CIS; most comparative clinical trials have found BCG immunotherapy to be significantly superior. Most therapeutic and prophylactic regimens are based on empirical use, not pharmacological data.

Prophylactic use consists of a single dose of mitomycin C or doxorubicin given as early as possible after transurethral resection of a bladder tumor (TURBT) – ideally within 6 hours of and no more than 24 hours after surgery. It has been shown to reduce the likelihood of further recurrences by about a third, presumably by killing cancer cells exfoliated during resection, which might otherwise be implanted and form new tumors.

Therapeutic use implies giving the drug to patients whose tumors cannot be completely resected surgically. While some studies have involved deliberately leaving a 'marker lesion' after resection to assess the efficacy of intravesical chemotherapy with good results, purely therapeutic use is uncommon, and usually ineffective. The combination of hyperthermia and mitomycin C in this context is being evaluated.

Adjunctive use involves a course of chemotherapy given to a patient at high risk of future recurrence in order to reduce the frequency of such events. Typically, this would involve six or eight instillations at weekly intervals, followed a few weeks later by cystoscopy to assess response.

Immunotherapy. Intravesical immunotherapy with BCG was first reported to be effective in decreasing papillary tumor recurrence by Morales and colleagues in 1976. Since then, it has been shown to be the most effective agent for prevention of recurrence and also to prevent tumor progression. BCG immunotherapy is also highly effective in CIS, resulting in complete remission of existing disease in up to 75–80% of those treated with repeated courses. The bacillus acts as a non-specific promoter of cellular immunity in the urothelium, causing activation of cytotoxic lymphocytes and release of various tumoricidal cytokines.

A disadvantage of BCG is its toxicity, which is greater than that of intravesical chemotherapy (Table 6.2). The toxicity may be substantial in patients who receive maintenance courses. For this reason, BCG immunotherapy is generally used for first-line treatment in only those with high-risk disease, and as a second-line therapy for those with lower-risk disease but continued recurrences after adequate intravesical chemotherapy. Some of the side effects of BCG may be prevented or decreased in severity through the prophylactic use of isoniazid in conjunction with each intravesical

TABLE 6.2

Complications of intravesical therapy

Complication	% of patients (number)	
	BCG (N = 2062)*	Chemotherapy
Fever	2.9 (75)	0
Granulomatous prostatitis	0.9 (23)	0
Pneumonitis/hepatitis	0.7 (18)	(3)[†]
Arthralgia	0.5 (12)	0
Hematuria	0.9 (24)	rare
Rash	0.3 (8)	9
Ureteral obstruction	0.3 (8)	(4)[†]
Epididymitis	0.4 (10)	0
Contracted bladder	0.2 (6)	0.1
Renal abscess	0.1 (2)	0
Sepsis	0.4 (10)	0
Cytopenia	0.1 (2)	(2)[†]

Between 60% and 80% of patients receiving BCG (bacille Calmette–Guérin) immunotherapy experience symptoms of cystitis and/or a mild influenzalike illness after each instillation. About 15% of patients report cystitis with mitomycin, but it is rarely necessary to stop treatment.
*Data from Lamm 1992. [†]Case reports.

treatment, but this is not yet standard practice. Deaths directly attributable to BCG have occurred, so it should be used only by urologists who have experience both in its administration and in the management of its side effects.

Given the success of BCG immunotherapy, several other immunotherapeutic agents have been investigated. The two for which the most clinical experience has been gathered are recombinant α-2b interferon (Intron A, Schering Plough) and bropirimine. Glashan reported complete response in 45% of patients with CIS following treatment with α-2b interferon, 100 mega units intravesically, delivered at weekly intervals for 12 weeks. Clinical studies using α-2b interferon as a single agent or in combination with BCG show some promise in patients who have failed to respond to BCG alone.

Like α-2b interferon, bropirimine has been shown to clear CIS in some patients who had failed previous BCG immunotherapy, but it is no longer used; the US Food and Drug Administration has not approved it because of uncertainties regarding its true anticancer efficacy, and some concerns about possible cardiotoxicity exist.

Surveillance for and treatment of extravesical recurrence

Surveillance for and early detection of recurrence are necessary. Before BCG immunotherapy became widespread, patients with high-risk disease generally underwent cystectomy and were at risk only of upper-tract recurrence (about 4–5%), or urethral recurrence (about 10%) if urethrectomy had not been performed. With the successful treatment of bladder tumors and CIS with BCG, more bladder recurrence and higher percentages of patients with upper-tract recurrence or progression have been reported. Administration of BCG to the upper tracts is difficult, but can be achieved by ureteric catheterization or the induction of vesicoureteric reflux with an indwelling double-J ureteric stent. Furthermore, newer technology in the form of small, flexible ureteroscopes allows some small papillary tumors of the upper urinary tract to be resected or laser fulgurated, thus treating the tumor without the need for nephroureterectomy.

Cystoscopy. Routine surveillance for superficial bladder tumors has generally consisted of quarterly cystoscopy for 2 years after an initial tumor, 6-monthly cystoscopy for an additional 2 years and annual cystoscopy thereafter if recurrent tumors have never been found. If recurrence is detected, the patient returns to the start of this schedule. As late recurrence can occur, lifelong surveillance is recommended, particularly for high-risk tumors. In the UK, patients with low- and intermediate-risk tumors are often discharged from follow-up after 10 years without recurrence. Such patients must be told, however, that any future episode of hematuria requires investigation. In the USA, lifelong surveillance is usually carried out, but no optimal schedule has been defined.

As mentioned previously, it has recently been determined that patients with a single, low-grade Ta tumor and a negative first-check cystoscopy can probably safely be permitted an immediate increase to a 9-month interval and then to annual follow-up if clear, as most recurrences in such patients will appear at the first surveillance cystoscopy.

Cytology. For patients with high-grade tumors, either papillary or CIS, voided or bladder wash cytology may be helpful as an adjunct to cystoscopy, especially for CIS. For low- or intermediate-grade (grade 1 or 2) tumors, the yield for cytology is low, and its routine use is therefore not recommended.

The test is usually performed at the time of cystoscopy, often with a saline wash of the bladder, because the sensitivity is higher thus than with a voided specimen. Results are not available for several days, and some expertise is required to perform the test and interpret the result.

Tumor markers. Several diagnostic tests have been studied recently. One second-generation test, the BTA stat test (a bladder tumor antigen test), has been shown in some series to be approximately twice as sensitive as cytology and is particularly effective for detecting the low- and intermediate-grade tumors that cytology misses. It takes only minutes to carry out and can be performed at

the time of cystoscopy. The BTA stat test has been available for
5–6 years in the USA and Europe, and some reports indicate that
it is more useful than cytology, although this opinion remains
controversial.

The BTA stat test is performed on unmodified (unbuffered) urine.
The method is similar to that of a pregnancy test, and the results
are available in 5 minutes. The BTA stat test detects a different
protein from that detected by the original BTA test, and the newer
test has a higher sensitivity, with specificity similar to that of the
original test.

A quantitative test, called BTA TRAK (Bard), which measures
the same protein as that detected by the BTA stat test, has also
been developed. The level of tumor-associated protein measured
by this system appears to correlate directly with increasing stage
and grade of tumor. This test may, therefore, allow serial follow-up
of patients and indicate response to therapy and prognosis for
recurring disease.

In the UK, surveillance cystoscopy is usually performed in the
outpatient setting with a flexible (diagnostic only) cystoscope. One
study showed that if flexible cystoscopy was omitted for patients
with a positive BTA stat test result and instead they were taken
directly to anesthesia and rigid cystoscopy for possible resection, the
cost savings were substantial, even allowing for a few with negative
results on rigid cystoscopy (i.e. false-positive BTA tests). Trials are
planned to determine whether the use of the BTA stat test can
reduce the use of cystoscopy.

A similar test that measures a nuclear matrix protein (NMP)
secreted by some bladder tumors has also been developed, called the
NMP22 assay. NMPs are involved in DNA replication and RNA
synthesis. They are released during cell death and can be detected in
the blood and in urine. NMP22 is present in transitional cell tumors
and can be detected by an immunoassay. The test has to be
performed in a laboratory.

Additionally, a number of molecular markers are being studied
for prediction of outcome. These markers include p53 and *RB1*
tumor suppressor genes.

The results of comparisons of various urinary markers for bladder cancer are shown in Table 4.1 (page 29). As yet, no single urinary test has sufficient sensitivity to exclude bladder cancer, and so no test can replace cystoscopy in the investigation of a patient with a suspected tumor. However, such tests may find a use in reducing the frequency of cystoscopies.

Key points – management of superficial disease

- Tumors can be classified into low-, intermediate- and high-risk tumors by means of pathology results, number of tumors at first cystoscopy and presence of recurrence at the 3-month review cystoscopy.
- Low-risk tumors may recur, but are unlikely to progress. They need cystoscopic follow-up only.
- Intermediate-risk tumors are more likely both to recur and to progress. A course of intravesical chemotherapy will reduce the risk of recurrence but not of progression.
- High-risk superficial bladder cancer is likely to recur and, unless adequately treated, to progress. It is fatal in up to 30% of patients. Intravesical BCG should be used, and if that is unsuccessful, early cystectomy should be carefully considered.
- As pathological interpretation is key to choosing the correct treatment, tumors reported as intermediate or high grade should be reviewed by an expert uropathologist.
- All new tumors should be discussed by a multidisciplinary team (MDT).
- The management of high-risk superficial cancer should be discussed by the specialist MDT.
- Cystectomies should be carried out at a center where at least 50 radical prostatectomies and cystectomies are performed each year.
- Patients should be fully involved in the choice of their treatment.

Key references

Bouffioux C, Kurth KH, Bono A et al. Intravesical adjuvant chemotherapy for superficial transitional cell bladder carcinoma: results of two European Organization for Research and Treatment of Cancer randomized trials with mitomycin C and doxorubicin comparing early versus delayed instillations and short-term versus long-term treatment. *J Urol* 1995;153:934–41.

Cookson MS, Sarosdy MF. Management of stage T1 superficial bladder cancer with intravesical BCG therapy. *J Urol* 1992;148:797–801.

Fitzpatrick JM. The natural history of superficial bladder carcinoma. *Semin Urol* 1993;11:127–36.

Fradet Y, Tardif M, Bourget L, Robert J. Clinical cancer progression in urinary bladder tumours evaluated by multiparameter flow cytometry with monoclonal antibodies. Laval University Urology Group. *Cancer Res* 1990;50:432–7.

Glashan RW. A randomized control study of intravesical α-2b-interferon in carcinoma in situ of the bladder. *J Urol* 1990;144:658–61.

Heney NM. Natural history of superficial bladder cancer. Prognostic features and long-term disease course. *Urol Clin North Am* 1992;19:429–33.

Herr HW, Wartinger DD, Fair WR, Oettgen HF. Bacillus Calmette–Guérin therapy for superficial bladder cancer: a 10-year follow-up. *J Urol* 1992;147:1020–3.

Hudson MA, Swanson PE, Nadler RB, Humphrey PA. p53 protein accumulation in superficial bladder cancer is a predictor of subsequent muscle invasion. *J Urol Pathol* 1994;2:307–18.

Jaske G and members of the EORTC-GU Group. Intravesical instillation of BCG in carcinoma in situ of the urinary bladder. In: Debruyne FMJ, Denis L, van der Meijden APM, eds. *BCG in Superficial Bladder Cancer: Proceedings of an EORTC Genitourinary Group Meeting.* New York: Alan R Liss, 1989:187–92.

Kurth KH, Schroeder FH, Tunn U et al. Adjuvant chemotherapy of superficial transitional cell bladder carcinoma: preliminary results of a European Organization for Research on Treatment of Cancer randomized trial comparing doxorubicin hydrochloride, ethoglucid and transurethral resection alone. *J Urol* 1984;132:258–62.

Lamm DL. Complications of bacillus Calmette–Guérin immunotherapy. *Urol Clin North Am* 1992;19: 565–72.

Lamm DL, Blumenstein BA, Crawford ED et al. A randomized trial of intravesical doxorubicin and immunotherapy with bacille Calmette–Guérin for transitional cell carcinoma of the bladder. *N Engl J Med* 1991;325:1205–9.

Malkowicz SB, Skinner DG. Development of upper tract carcinoma after cystectomy for bladder cancer. *Urology* 1990;36: 20–2.

Morales A, Eidinger D, Bruce AW. Adjuvant immunotherapy with BCG in recurrent superficial bladder cancer. In: Lamoureux G, Turcotte R, Portelance V, eds. *BCG in Cancer Immunotherapy*. New York: Grune & Stratton, 1976:247–52.

Nadler RB, Catalona WJ, Hudson MA, Ratliff TL. Durability of the tumor-free response for intravesical bacillus Calmette–Guérin therapy. *J Urol* 1994;152:367–73.

National Institute for Clinical Excellence (UK). *Improving Outcomes in Urological Cancers.* London: NICE, 2002. www.nice.org.uk/pdf/Urological_Manual.pdf

Newling D. Intravesical therapy in the management of superficial transitional cell carcinoma of the bladder: the experience of the EORTC group. *Br J Cancer* 1990; 61:497–9.

Okamura T, Tozawa K, Yamada Y et al. Clinicopathological evaluation of repeated courses of intravesical bacillus Calmette–Guérin instillation for preventing recurrence of initially resistant superficial bladder cancer. *J Urol* 1996;156:967–71.

Pagano F, Garbeglio A, Milani C et al. Prognosis of bladder cancer. I. Risk factors in superficial transitional cell carcinoma. *Eur Urol* 1987;13:145–9.

Sarosdy MF, Hudson MA, Ellis WJ et al. Improved detection of recurrent bladder cancer using the BARD BTA stat Test. *Urology* 1997;50:349–53.

Sarosdy MF, Lowe BA, Schellhammer PF et al. Oral bropirimine immunotherapy of carcinoma in situ of the bladder: results of a phase II trial. *Urology* 1996;48:21–7.

Sarosdy MF, deVere White RW, Soloway MS et al. Results of a multicenter trial using the BTA test to monitor for and diagnose recurrent bladder cancer. *J Urol* 1995;154: 379–83.

Sarosdy MF. Principles of intravesical chemotherapy and immunotherapy. *Urol Clin North Am* 1992;19: 509–19.

Schmeller NT, Hofstetter AG. Laser treatment of ureteral tumors. *J Urol* 1989;141:840–3.

Soloway MS, Briggman JV, Carpinito GA et al. Use of a new tumour marker, urinary NMP-22, in the detection of occult or rapidly recurring transitional cell carcinoma of the urinary tract following surgical treatment. *J Urol* 1996;156:363–7.

Vegt PD, Witjes JA, Witjes WP et al. A randomized study of intravesical mitomycin C, bacillus Calmette–Guérin Tice and bacillus Calmette-Guérin RIVM treatment in pTa–pT1 papillary carcinoma and carcinoma in situ of the bladder. *J Urol* 1995;153:929–33.

Muscle invasion indicates a poor prognosis in bladder cancer, with overall survival rates of around 50% at 5 years. Radical treatment is necessary if the patient is to be offered a chance of cure. There are two mainstays of treatment:
- surgical removal of the bladder (cystectomy)
- radiotherapy.

These can be used alone or in combination.

Staging of invasive disease

Before the treatment for an individual is decided, as much information as possible must be obtained about the extent of the disease. In patients with T2/T3N0M0 disease, treatment should be offered with curative intent. If the tumor is T2/T3N1M0, cure is less likely; in the case of N2 or M1 disease, palliation is the most common aim, although occasional patients may be cured by the combination of neoadjuvant, or front-line, intravenous chemotherapy followed by cystectomy. Some patients will have T4 tumors because of prostatic involvement, but, if these are N0/M0, may still be cured. A number of investigations can be carried out to identify the stage and grade of the tumor.

Cystoscopy and biopsy with bimanual examination. During cystoscopy in a patient with suspected invasive disease, biopsies should be taken with a resectoscope, sufficiently deep to include muscle, in order to allow accurate histological staging and grading of the tumor. A 'cold cup' biopsy of the tumor site after resection should ensure the presence of muscle. At the end of the cystoscopy, with the bladder empty and the patient relaxed, the bladder is palpated bimanually with a finger in the rectum (in men) or vagina (in women) and suprapubic pressure applied with the other hand. The presence of a palpable thickening or mass in the bladder wall suggests invasive disease. Clinical staging can thus be established.

CT scanning is performed with intravenous, oral and rectal contrast to establish the degree of invasion of the tumor into the bladder and perivesical tissues (Figure 7.1), as well as to identify lymphadenopathy, ureteric obstruction or liver or pulmonary metastases. The procedure is usually accurate in identifying extravesical extension of the tumor, but scarring from previous transurethral resections of the tumor can sometimes cause problems with diagnosis. Caution should be exercised when interpreting a CT scan shortly after resection of a bladder tumor, since the post-resection artifact can resemble invasive disease.

MRI can provide better images of the pelvic organs and allow more accurate assessment of the extent of invasion by the tumor than CT scanning (Figure 7.2).

Chest radiography. If CT scanning of the chest has not been performed, a chest radiograph is needed to exclude pulmonary metastases.

Bone scanning. While not a routine part of the staging investigation, a bone scan should be obtained if there are any symptoms that might suggest metastasis to bone, or if the serum alkaline phosphatase level is elevated.

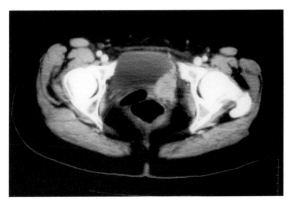

Figure 7.1 CT scan of the pelvic area in a patient with invasive bladder cancer, indicating penetration of the tumor into the perivesical fat.

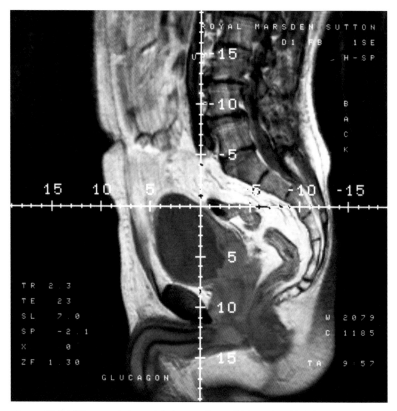

Figure 7.2 MRI scan of the pelvis in a patient with invasive bladder cancer.

Treatment options

Several treatment options exist for patients with muscle-invasive bladder cancer (Table 7.1).

Primary radiotherapy was once the most common first-line treatment offered to patients with invasive bladder cancer in the UK, though it has now been overtaken by primary cystectomy.

Radiotherapy is given in a variety of ways (Figure 7.3), with changes in the fractionation (the way the total dose is divided) designed to achieve maximum effect on the tumor while minimizing side effects. Typically, treatment is given during a series of outpatient visits over a 6- or 7-week period. The field covered by the radiation will include the bladder, prostate and pelvic

TABLE 7.1

Treatment options for muscle-invasive bladder cancer

- Radiotherapy
- Radical surgery (with or without neoadjuvant chemotherapy)
  - cystectomy with ileal conduit urinary diversion
  - cystectomy with orthotopic bladder reconstruction
  - cystectomy with continent urinary diversion
- Chemoradiation
- Preoperative radiotherapy with subsequent cystectomy (rarely used now)

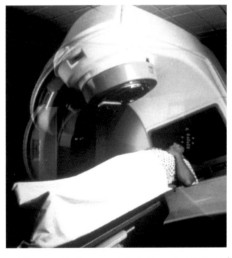

Figure 7.3 External-beam radiotherapy with a linear accelerator for carcinoma of the bladder.

lymph nodes, with doses of 68–70 Gy delivered to the tumor and surrounding tissue. Inevitably, some radiation damage will occur in neighboring structures, in particular the rectum, small bowel and ureters.

Early side effects of radiotherapy include skin, bowel and bladder sensitivity, nausea and tiredness. Late effects include reduction in bladder capacity, increased frequency of bowel movements, hematuria and rectal bleeding. Occasionally, these effects can be severe and may even require surgical intervention. With good planning, careful dosimetry and supervision of treatment to allow dose alteration if side effects develop, radiotherapy is usually well tolerated.

Radical surgery. In the USA, Australia, Canada and some European countries, patients are likely to be offered surgery as the initial treatment for non-metastatic invasive bladder cancer. More recently, in the UK, primary cystectomy has also largely superseded radiotherapy.

The development of techniques avoiding ileal conduit diversion ('a bag') has helped to make surgery a more attractive option.

Cystectomy. The mainstay of surgical treatment of invasive bladder cancer is removal of the bladder. As the whole of the urothelium has been exposed to whatever carcinogen initiated the cancer, the urethra must also be considered to be at risk of developing a tumor. For this reason, cystectomy is usually combined with total prostatectomy and sometimes urethrectomy (Figure 7.4). If on biopsy there is no evidence of tumor in the prostatic urethra in men, or in the bladder neck in women, and if the bladder tumor is not associated with extensive CIS, the urethra may be preserved, allowing construction of a new bladder from intestine.

The operation is performed under general anesthesia via a transperitoneal approach. The lymph nodes draining the bladder are excised, the peritoneum over the bladder is divided and a plane between the bladder and the rectum is developed. The ureters are identified and divided, and the lateral pedicles of the bladder with its three main arteries are ligated and divided. The prostate is mobilized, and if a new bladder is to be made, the urethra is divided at the apex of the prostate in men, or the bladder neck in women. If a cystoprostatectomy and urethrectomy is being performed, the urethra is mobilized through a perineal incision and removed en bloc with the bladder and, in men, the prostate, or, in women, a strip of the anterior wall of the vagina.

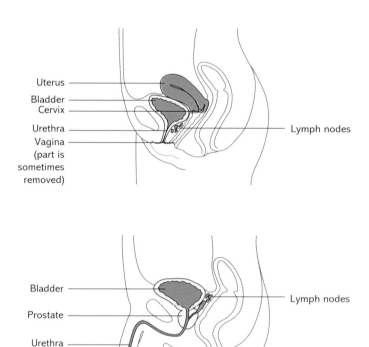

Uterus
Bladder
Cervix
Urethra
Vagina
(part is
sometimes
removed)
Lymph nodes

Bladder
Prostate
Urethra
(not always
removed)
Lymph nodes

Figure 7.4 Cystectomy in women and men: the shaded parts are removed.

Reconstruction after cystectomy. Following cystectomy, some means of diverting the flow of urine from the ureters must be employed. Several techniques are possible, each with its own advantages and disadvantages. Not all will be appropriate for every patient. Studies have shown that techniques avoiding an incontinent stoma provide some benefits in quality of life, but perhaps the best way to achieve a satisfactory outcome – that is, an outcome that satisfies the patient – is to ensure that he or she is fully informed and involved in the choice of reconstruction.

Ileal loop (conduit). The traditional procedure once offered to most patients involves isolating a loop of ileum attached to its vascular pedicle, anastomosing the ureters to one end of the loop and bringing the other end out of the abdominal wall as a stoma (an ileal conduit urinary diversion; Figure 7.5).

While this is the simplest reconstruction, many patients find the idea of living with a bag to collect urine unacceptable, so other forms of diversion are increasingly being utilized.

Orthotopic bladder reconstruction. It is possible to create a new bladder from intestinal segments using one of a variety of

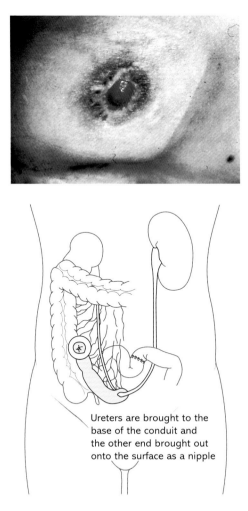

Ureters are brought to the base of the conduit and the other end brought out onto the surface as a nipple

Figure 7.5 An ileal conduit urinary diversion.

techniques. When this can be done without compromising the chance of cure, and when the patient is fit enough to withstand the extra surgery involved, the option of avoiding a urostomy is very attractive to the patient.

If a neobladder is to be fashioned, the dissection around the junction between the urethra and the bladder neck in women, or the prostate in men, needs to be conducted with great care to preserve the distal sphincter. The new bladder can be made from small bowel, the ileocecal segment or large bowel. The bowel is isolated on its vascular pedicle, opened along the antimesenteric border and sutured to create a pouch with a capacity of 400–800 mL (Figure 7.6). The ureters are anastomosed to the posterosuperior aspect of the pouch, and an anastomosis is created between the most dependent part of the pouch and the urethral stump. This procedure takes longer than a standard cystectomy, and involves a longer hospital stay. It can be offered to women as well as men, despite earlier concerns about continence.

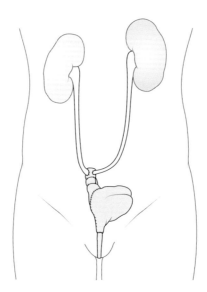

Figure 7.6 A neobladder allows the patient to pass urine as normal during the day, though leakage may occur at night.

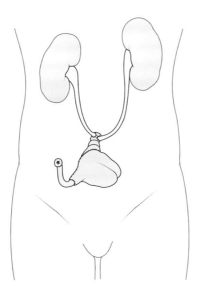

Figure 7.7 With a continent stoma, urine is drained using a catheter passed through the stoma and into the pouch.

Creation of a continent stoma. In patients who are very keen to avoid a stoma draining into a bag, but in whom orthotopic reconstruction is not feasible (e.g. because of the presence of CIS in the distal prostatic urethra, or when the urethra has extensive stricture disease), a pouch can be made as described above. It is then brought to the surface using a continent, catheterizable stoma (Figure 7.7). The catheterizable stoma can be constructed from the appendix, tunneled into the wall of the pouch so as to create a flap-valve effect. This allows passage of a catheter to empty the pouch periodically, while maintaining continence between these self-catheterizations.

Rectosigmoid (Mainz-2) pouch. Another form of diversion suitable for construction when the urethra has to be sacrificed is the Mainz-2 pouch. The sigmoid colon and rectum are detubularized to create a low-pressure reservoir to which the ureters are joined (Figure 7.8). The urine is then passed via the anus.

Salvage cystectomy. When a recurrent tumor is found in the bladder after full-dose radiotherapy, salvage cystectomy may be

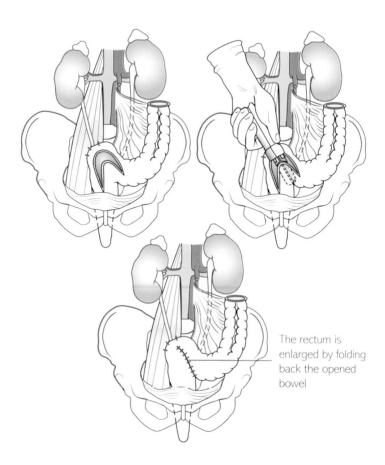

The rectum is enlarged by folding back the opened bowel

Figure 7.8 The rectosigmoid (Mainz-2) pouch.

attempted so long as there is no evidence of distant metastasis. It must be emphasized that this is technically difficult surgery, as the tissues are damaged after radiotherapy, with extensive scarring. Nevertheless, if the lymph nodes are negative and staging for metastatic deposits is negative, patients may be cured by salvage cystectomy. In one current strategy for bladder preservation, the group at the Massachusetts General Hospital administers chemoradiation in a dose of 40–45 Gy and then reassesses the tumor; in patients with residual viable cancer at this point, early salvage cystectomy is implemented before the development of extensive scarring. In this fashion, these investigators attempt to maximize the chance of bladder preservation without sacrificing the potential for cure by cystectomy.

Chemotherapy. In the past 20 years, the role of systemic chemotherapy in the treatment of invasive bladder cancer has been explored. Since the majority of failures of therapy are a result of systemic relapse rather than local failure, it was logical to consider the possibility that cytotoxic agents, delivered early, might eradicate occult metastases. Chemotherapy has been delivered in several ways:
• before definitive local treatment (so-called preemptive or neoadjuvant chemotherapy)
• synchronously with radiotherapy (chemoradiation)
• after completion of definitive radiotherapy or surgery (adjuvant chemotherapy).

Neoadjuvant (preemptive) chemotherapy was first studied in trials of single-agent regimens. Although tumor reduction was observed, no survival benefit was demonstrated in randomized trials. However, a series of randomized trials has demonstrated a survival benefit from neoadjuvant combination chemotherapy. For example, a collaborative trial of the Medical Research Council (UK) and the European Organisation for Research and Treatment of Cancer (EORTC), which compared definitive local treatment alone with initial cisplatin–methotrexate–vinblastine (CMV) chemotherapy followed by definitive local treatment (radiation or cystectomy), identified a 5–6% survival benefit for the CMV group. The North American Intergroup found a 7% survival benefit achieved by neoadjuvant methotrexate–vinblastine–doxorubicin–cisplatin (the MVAC regimen) before radical cystectomy, and this difference was statistically significant. Other studies have shown similar results, although it is noted that the Radiation Therapy Oncology Group (RTOG) in the USA did not identify any survival benefit from neoadjuvant CMV chemotherapy prior to chemoradiation with single-agent cisplatin. A meta-analysis has confirmed that single-agent neoadjuvant

63

chemotherapy is ineffective, but that combination neoadjuvant chemotherapy yields a small, but statistically significant, survival benefit before local therapy.

Chemoradiation. Initial studies of chemoradiation, using radiotherapy in association with single cytotoxic agents or combination chemotherapy regimens, have shown significant tumor reduction and have suggested the possibility of improved survival compared with historical data (a flawed assessment due to statistical methodology). Only one randomized trial, conducted by the National Cancer Institute of Canada, has assessed the utility of chemoradiation and demonstrated statistically improved local control compared with radiotherapy alone. This trial did not identify any statistically significant improvement in survival, although it was not designed as a study with survival as a primary endpoint. It has been reasoned that chemoradiation is useful in achieving better local control than radiotherapy alone, and that more effective systemic therapy should be developed to achieve a survival benefit (given that most relapses are systemic).

Adjuvant chemotherapy. To date, only three randomized trials have assessed the usefulness of adjuvant chemotherapy after cystectomy for invasive bladder cancer. These trials studied contemporary regimens, such as cyclophosphamide–doxorubicin–cisplatin (CAP), CMV and MVAC. The studies were substantially flawed in design and/or execution, but did suggest a trend in favor of improved survival (not achieving statistical significance). In common clinical practice in North America, there is an increasing tendency to deliver adjuvant MVAC or CMV chemotherapy for node-positive TCC after cystectomy, but we emphasize that the benefit of this approach has not been proved in well-structured clinical trials. For this reason, an international collaboration between the EORTC and other groups attempted to assess the true value of adjuvant MVAC chemotherapy after completion of definitive local treatment. However, accrual has been very low and it seems likely that this study will close before completion of planned accrual.

Treatment outcomes

The results of radiotherapy or surgery depend on the grade and stage of the tumor. Overall 5-year survival rates for N0 patients following cystectomy are:

- pT2 disease: 60–80%
- pT3a disease: 50–70%
- pT3b disease: 30–60%.

Approximately 50% of all patients undergoing 'curative' treatment for bladder cancer will develop metastatic disease and die within 2–3 years of treatment.

In the UK, it was believed in the past that survival rates with radiotherapy and cystectomy were similar. A recent meta-analysis has shown a survival benefit for surgery; however, as exact pathological staging of the tumor and lymph nodes is not available for patients treated with radiotherapy, direct comparisons are difficult. Well-designed randomized clinical comparisons of these modalities are not available.

In North America, the prevalent view is that cystectomy yields superior long-term survival. While the comparisons of surgically staged and clinically staged cases have serious inherent selection bias, there are no radiation series that yield cure rates as high as those reported for patients with deeply invasive and node-positive bladder cancer treated by cystectomy by Stein and colleagues from the University of Southern California.

With the development of continent ileostomies and neobladders, the quality-of-life discrepancies between radical surgery and radiotherapy have been reduced significantly. This applies particularly to the avoidance of an ileostomy bag and the ability to regain continence (see below).

Quality of life following surgery

The prime concern of most patients with bladder cancer is to be cured of the disease. Apart from concerns about death, symptoms such as severe frequency, dysuria, urgency, hematuria and bladder pain may be sufficient to justify cystectomy even if cure is not possible. Relief of these symptoms represents a great improvement in a patient's quality of life.

The negative effects of cystectomy must be carefully explained to patients prior to embarking on surgery. In men, ejaculation will not occur, and those in whom erections are maintained will experience altered sensation at orgasm. Erectile failure is likely, even if attempts are made to spare the nerve supply to the corpora cavernosa, which passes close to the prostate; 50–70% of men will be impotent after cystectomy. In women, a conventional cystectomy includes hysterectomy and excision of the anterior vaginal wall, which will narrow the vagina and may cause dyspareunia. The operation can be modified in sexually active women to preserve vaginal volume. The patient must learn to cope with a urostomy, unless a bladder reconstruction or a continent diversion has been constructed.

While orthotopic bladder reconstruction eliminates the need for a stoma, the new bladder does not function like a normal one, and brings problems of its own, such as incontinence. With careful attention to technique, diurnal continence rates of 85% have been achieved. Most patients who experience problems do so at night. Men can use a condom drainage system; women may be dependent on incontinence pads. Another problem experienced is inadequate emptying. Most patients learn how to empty their bladder by relaxing the sphincter and increasing intra-abdominal pressure. If this does not achieve satisfactory results, intermittent self-catheterization may be necessary. A continent urinary diversion suffers from the same problems as a neobladder, except that difficulties with the catheterizable stoma replace problems with the sphincter mechanism.

As the bowel segment secretes mucus, and as emptying may not always be complete, UTIs are more likely in cystectomy patients. Providing the ureters have been implanted with an antireflux technique, ascending infection should not be a problem.

In spite of the many potential difficulties with continent diversions or orthotopic bladder replacement, these techniques offer a significant psychological benefit to patients undergoing cystectomy.

Key points – management of muscle-invasive disease

- Options for treatment of muscle-invasive bladder cancer are cystectomy, radiotherapy or chemoradiation.
- New techniques for bladder reconstruction can prevent the need for a 'bag' in most patients.
- Evidence from good-quality randomized trials to identify relative cure rates of these different options is lacking, although randomized trials have shown that neoadjuvant chemotherapy (CMV or MVAC) plus cystectomy improve long-term survival compared with cystectomy alone.
- Cure rates of 60–80% can be achieved in tumors confined to the detrusor muscle.
- Failure of therapy is usually due to micrometastatic disease present but undetectable at the time of initial therapy. Recent studies suggest that neoadjuvant chemotherapy may improve survival by eradicating micrometastases.
- The overall cure rate remains low, as many patients present with locally advanced disease.

Quality of life following radiotherapy

The obvious benefit of treatment with radiotherapy is the potential for retention of the natural bladder without the need for a stoma or reconstruction. As a result, control of micturition is usually excellent, and fewer than 50–60% of male patients are impotent. In patients with a previous history of recurrent superficial bladder cancer (with repeated transurethral resections of bladder tumors, or TURBTs), there is an increased risk of postradiation bladder symptoms. These include the features of a contracted or scarred bladder, namely reduced bladder capacity and symptoms of cystitis, with the need for repeated micturition, which is especially irritating for the patient during the hours of sleep. The higher the dose of radiotherapy, the greater the prevalence of symptoms and side effects, especially above doses of 68–70 Gy. If chemoradiation is used, the application of cytotoxics with radiosensitizing potential, such as cisplatin, 5-fluorouracil, paclitaxel and gemcitabine, is likely to increase the level of irritative symptoms. Nevertheless, one of us has previously demonstrated excellent quality of life in patients (who have not undergone repeated TURBT) treated with single-agent cisplatin or CMV and radiotherapy.

Key references

Advanced Bladder Cancer Meta-analysis Collaboration. Neoadjuvant chemotherapy in invasive bladder cancer: a systematic review and meta-analysis. *Lancet* 2003;361:1922–3.

Bloom H, Hendry W, Wallace D et al. Treatment of T3 bladder cancer: controlled trial of preoperative radiotherapy and radical cystectomy versus radical radiotherapy. Second report and review. *Br J Urol* 1982;54:136–42.

Fossa S, Woehre H, Aass N et al. Definitive radiation therapy of muscle invasive bladder cancer: a retrospective review of 317 patients. *Cancer* 1993;72:3036–45.

Grossman HB, Natale RB, Tangen CM et al. Neoadjuvant chemotherapy plus cystectomy compared with cystectomy alone for locally advanced bladder cancer. *N Engl J Med* 2003;349:859–66.

National Institute for Clinical Excellence (UK). *Improving Outcomes in Urological Cancers.* London: NICE, 2002. www.nice.org.uk/pdf/Urological_Manual.pdf

Raghavan D, Quinn D, Skinner DG, Stein JP. Surgery and adjunctive chemotherapy for invasive bladder cancer. *Surg Oncol* 2002;11:55–63.

Raghavan D, Shipley WU, Hall RR, Richie JP. Biology and management of invasive bladder cancer. In: Raghavan D, Scher H, Leibel S, Lange P, eds. *Principles and Practice of Genitourinary Oncology.* Philadelphia: JB Lippincott, 1997:281–98.

Stein JP, Lieskovsky G, Cote R et al. Radical cystectomy in the treatment of invasive bladder cancer: long-term results in 1054 patients. *J Clin Oncol* 2001;19:666–75.

Patients with tumors extending outside the limits that can be treated by radiotherapy or removed surgically generally have a poor prognosis, although survival has increased from the 3–6 months it averaged in the period from 1950 to 1970 (depending on the extent of the disease). Only 10–20% of patients with T4 disease will survive 5 years, and of those with known metastatic tumors, 50% will die within 18 months. The management of these patients must be directed to improving quality of life as much as attempting to increase longevity.

Treatment

The development of multiagent combination chemotherapy regimens has greatly improved response rates to treatment and survival of patients with advanced and metastatic bladder cancer. The CMV and MVAC regimens, comprising cisplatin, methotrexate and vinblastine, with or without doxorubicin, yielded objective response rates of around 50–70% in some series, and the median survival approached 12 months. An international randomized clinical trial compared single-agent cisplatin with the MVAC regimen and showed a clear survival benefit, with a median survival for MVAC of about 12 months and a 25–30% survival at 3–5 years. When cisplatin alone was used, the median survival was 8 months and the survival rate at 3–5 years was only 10%. An important finding of the trial was that more than two-thirds of patients experienced sustained improvement in symptoms, and sites of response included osseous and hepatic metastases. A late analysis at 7 years, published in 1997, showed that most of the patients in this trial had died, either of intercurrent disease or malignancy; however, more than 80% of the survivors were in the MVAC-treated group. More recent reports suggest that the median survival when the MVAC regimen is used is around 18 months; this probably represents 'stage migration', that is, treatment of patients with smaller-volume metastatic disease, consequent upon increased use of CT and MRI scans in the follow-up of patients treated by radiotherapy or cystectomy.

This is a highly toxic regimen, and it is not a panacea for advanced bladder cancer, especially since the regimen is relatively inactive in patients with advanced squamous cell carcinoma and adenocarcinoma.

In recent years, a series of novel cytotoxics, including ifosfamide, paclitaxel, docetaxel and gemcitabine, have been assessed in the management of advanced disease. Several doublets, often combining one of these agents with cisplatin, have shown high levels of activity with much less toxicity than the MVAC regimen. One of us has previously shown that gemcitabine achieves objective responses in around 30% of patients when used as a single agent, and in up to 50% of cases when combined with cisplatin. A randomized trial has shown that the MVAC regimen and the gemcitabine–cisplatin combination have very similar activities, but that the latter is much less toxic. Other regimens, such as the combination of ifosfamide, cisplatin and paclitaxel, are also active, with objective response rates of 50–80%, depending on the nature of metastatic disease.

An international randomized trial recently compared the utility of gemcitabine–cisplatin versus gemcitabine–cisplatin–paclitaxel, although results are not yet available, and other groups are assessing the role of non-cross-resistant regimens, such as the alternating combination of ifosfamide–paclitaxel–cisplatin and doxorubicin–gemcitabine. Eventually, these trials will identify a new standard of care, although current practice has defined gemcitabine–cisplatin as the replacement for the MVAC regimen for patients with metastatic disease (Table 8.1).

Palliation

The role of chemotherapy in the palliation of advanced bladder cancer depends completely on the context – specifically, the age, performance status, distribution of disease, presence of symptoms and nature of previous therapy. In the patient who has received

TABLE 8.1

Typical outcomes from contemporary chemotherapy regimens

Regimen	Typical response rate (%)	Median survival (months)
MVAC	30–70	12–18
GC	50–65	12–15
GCT	85	~24
GCaT	70	~15
TCa	50–60	~9
TC	50–70	~12
ITC	68–79	~18

A, doxorubicin; C, cisplatin; Ca, carboplatin; G, gemcitabine; I, ifosfamide; M, methotrexate; T, paclitaxel; V, vinblastine.

various types of chemotherapy, the respective gains and drawbacks of further cytotoxics must be considered very carefully. However, with the availability of less toxic and modestly effective second-line regimens, the decision process has become more complex. It thus behooves the clinician to be completely familiar with the recent literature on this topic.

Symptoms requiring palliation can be local or distant.

Progression of local disease. Irritative voiding symptoms, such as urgency, frequency, dysuria and strangury, can cause extreme discomfort. Hematuria may be sufficient to require regular blood transfusions and may even be life-threatening. Clot retention of urine may require repeated visits to the hospital for emergency treatment.

It is always worth excluding a UTI, which is more likely to develop in a patient with necrotic tumor than others. Treatment may reduce irritative symptoms from an infection.

The treatment of tumor-related hematuria can be very difficult. Possible treatment options are outlined in Table 8.2. Palliative

TABLE 8.2

Treatment of hematuria in metastatic bladder cancer

- Transurethral resection and fulguration, if tumor still present
- Palliative irradiation of the bladder, if radiotherapy not used previously
- Palliative chemotherapy with/without forced hydration
- Irrigation with alum, if above techniques unsuccessful
- Palliative simple cystectomy, if there is minimal metastatic disease and the patient is relatively fit, or urinary diversion
- Formalin instillation, if all else fails

radiotherapy or cystoscopy and transurethral resection of a focal area of tumor tissue may improve the patient's level of comfort substantially. Similarly, it is not uncommon to see dramatic improvement in symptoms over a few days after the initial administration of systemic cisplatin-containing chemotherapy with forced hydration and diuresis; this can be seen with single-agent cisplatin, gemcitabine–cisplatin or the MVAC regimen. For more resistant cases, alum can be administered over 24–48 hours as a 5% solution via a three-way irrigating catheter. It is non-toxic and has little, if any, effect on bladder capacity.

Formalin is more effective at stopping bleeding but is more hazardous. It is used as a 4% solution, instilled into the bladder for 15 minutes and then drained through a catheter. The procedure requires general anesthesia as it is very painful. Following treatment, bladder capacity may be drastically reduced, causing severe frequency of urination or incontinence; reflux into the kidneys may cause renal failure. For these reasons, formalin instillation is rarely used.

Palliative cystectomy may be justified in the highly symptomatic patient with minimal metastatic disease, provided the patient is reasonably fit. In the patient with more extensive metastatic disease, urinary diversion may reduce the discomfort associated with urinary flow and bladder spasm in this setting.

Progression of distant symptoms. Sadly, in spite of the best efforts of surgeons and radiotherapists, most patients with invasive bladder cancer will die of their disease. It is important that the doctors caring for these patients be aware of how much impact the quality of life has, not just on the patients, but on relatives and friends as well. Whatever treatment is planned, patients and next of kin should be fully involved in the decision-making process. It must be made clear that the aim of treatment is palliation and not cure, and full explanation must be given of what can be expected.

Bone metastases. Bone pain from metastases may be severe and distressing in its own right. Even more suffering may be caused if the metastasis involves a long bone and pathological fracture ensues. Cord compression from vertebral collapse or rapidly expanding dural deposits is one of the most severe effects of metastasis. Once it is established, there is little chance of recovery of motor or sensory function, and the patient is likely to end life in a wheelchair, incontinent of urine and feces. For this reason, any symptoms suggesting early cord compression (paresthesia in the legs, loss of power, or loss of bladder or bowel control) in a patient with malignant disease must be treated as a medical emergency. Immediate treatment with dexamethasone, followed by surgical decompression or radiotherapy, may prevent progression to paraplegia.

Uremia, characterized by anorexia, malaise, an unpleasant taste in the mouth and occasionally oliguria, may be due to ureteric obstruction. The decision to treat or not to treat renal failure in the presence of incurable malignancy is not an easy one. A patient who is otherwise fairly free of symptoms may request relief of the obstruction. Usually, if the tumor has not yet been treated with the best available therapy, then nephrostomy drainage or internal ureteric stenting is appropriate. However, in patients whose tumor has advanced in spite of treatment, renal failure may offer a relatively rapid and pain-free escape from a terminal illness. The pros and cons of this decision should be carefully explained to the patient and relatives.

73

Other systemic symptoms, such as a cough from pulmonary deposits, malignant pleural effusion, capsular pain or jaundice from liver metastases and anemia as a result of bone marrow replacement, are all common in advanced metastatic bladder cancer. The treatment of these symptoms is best managed in conjunction with a palliative care team, who may be able to offer drug treatment to relieve specific symptoms, as well as moral and psychological support for patients and their carers.

Transfusion may be needed if anemia causes symptoms, although the benefit is short-lived and repeated transfusions may be necessary. If the anemia is due to iron deficiency from continuing hematuria, iron supplements are indicated. Often, though, the anemia is due to marrow replacement by tumor, and supplements are contraindicated.

Pain is perhaps the least well managed aspect of palliative care. It is essential that the physician takes an adequate pain history and applies a detailed knowledge of the principals of pain management. The physician should be familiar with the graduated pain scale and the optimal use of increasing levels of analgesia, including non-steroidal anti-inflammatory medications, narcotic analgesics (in particular, the depot preparations), coanalgesics and devices such as epidural catheters and regional blocks. Pain should be regarded as a medical emergency, and adequate analgesia must be provided at once. Delaying narcotic analgesia for severe pain 'until it is really needed' is an outmoded and cruel concept, and has no place in current management.

When the patient is suffering from pain that is hard to control, the aid of a palliative care team should be enlisted, even when an attempt at palliation over several months in association with radiotherapy or chemotherapy is envisaged. All centers treating patients with malignant disease should have strong links with such a team, and local guidelines should exist regarding the stage at which patients should be referred.

There is much to be said for the early introduction of palliative care specialists. They have special skills in helping patients come to terms with the knowledge that their life expectancy is limited. Even if no direct intervention is needed following the first meeting, it will reassure the patient to know that they are available, and will inspire confidence when the time comes to call on their services. This support can often allow the patient to remain at home during most or all of the terminal illness. The palliative care team will work closely with the patient's primary care physician to achieve this.

In addition to the optimum use of opiate analgesics, the palliative care team may be able to offer nerve blocks, epidural injections, transepidermal nerve stimulation or acupuncture to provide pain relief. Other troublesome symptoms such as nausea, itching, dyspnea and depression can often be helped by appropriate drug therapy.

Although bone pain can be controlled initially with non-steroidal anti-inflammatory drugs, the possibility of pathological fractures must be borne in mind, especially if the spine or long bones are involved. Radiotherapy is very effective in relieving bone pain and is usually given to the affected area in one or two fractions. If several bones are involved (Figure 8.1), strontium-90 (Metastron) may be given intravenously as a single bolus dose. It is taken up selectively by areas of increased bone turnover, thereby irradiating the metastatic deposits in the skeleton. Radiotherapy may also be given to soft tissue deposits if they are causing pain or threatening compression of vital structures.

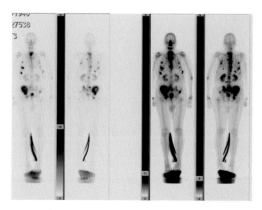

Figure 8.1 Bone scan showing multiple 'hot spots' corresponding to bony secondary deposits from carcinoma of the bladder.

Key points – management of advanced and metastatic disease

- Some patients with metastatic disease, especially if it is limited to lymph nodes and soft tissues, may achieve cure or sustained palliation (the latter lasting for 3–5 years in up to 25% of cases).
- The management of advanced and metastatic disease should involve a team comprising clinical oncologists, surgeons, radiation oncologists and palliative care physicians.
- The aim of treatment is to optimize the patient's quality of life and to prolong life when possible.
- The careful planning of surgical, radiotherapeutic, chemotherapeutic and palliative care inputs in a patient's last few months can make the difference between a dignified and pain-free death or several months of miserable existence.

Key references

Harrison P. Update on pain management for advanced genitourinary cancer. *J Urol* 2001;165:1849–58.

National Institute for Clinical Excellence (UK). *Improving Outcomes in Urological Cancers.* London: NICE, 2002. www.nice.org.uk/pdf/Urological_Manual.pdf

Raghavan D. Progress in the chemotherapy of metastatic cancer of the urinary tract. *Cancer* 2003;97(8 suppl):2050–5.

Raghavan D. Molecular targeting and pharmacogenomics in the management of advanced bladder cancer. *Cancer* 2003;97(8 suppl): 2083–9.

Schwartz CB, Bekirov H, Melman A. Urothelial tumors of upper tract following treatment of primary bladder transitional cell carcinoma. *Urology* 1992;40:509–11.

Sternberg CN, Yagoda A, Scher HI. Methotrexate, vinblastine, doxorubicin, and cisplatin for advanced transitional cell carcinoma of the urothelium: efficacy and patterns of response and relapse. *Cancer* 1989;64:2448–58.

The mortality and morbidity of bladder cancer could be reduced by:
- disease prevention
- earlier diagnosis
- better treatment of high-risk superficial disease
- improvements in existing therapies
- development of new treatments.

Prevention

A number of bladder carcinogens have been identified. The recognition of the carcinogenic properties of aniline dyes and aromatic amines used in industrial processes has led to a ban on these agents. The most common carcinogen involved in bladder cancer – cigarette smoke – has escaped such a fate. Smoking is probably responsible for 30–40% of cases of bladder cancer, and the association between bladder cancer and smoking is stronger than that for lung cancer. In patients with superficial tumors, the recurrence rate is higher and the chance of progression to invasive disease is greater in those who continue to smoke. It follows that the single greatest preventive measure possible would be to eliminate cigarette smoking. As this is politically unacceptable, we must continue to inform the public of the health hazards of this practice.

Environmental causes such as atmospheric pollution may play a significant role in the etiology of bladder cancer – diesel fumes and particulates lead to a higher incidence in urban areas. Initiatives to reduce this pollution could have a beneficial effect on rates of bladder cancer.

One of the more common causes of bladder cancer worldwide is infection with *Schistosoma haematobium*. Public health measures to eliminate schistosomiasis have been hindered in some countries by economic difficulties and political uncertainty.

Apart from the avoidance of known carcinogens, there is little else that can be done to prevent bladder cancer at present.

Earlier diagnosis

Screening. The increased use of urine dipstick testing for hematuria may lead to detection of some tumors at an earlier stage. Populations at high risk because of industrial exposure are routinely screened by this method. Voided urine cytology is not sufficiently sensitive to be used for routine screening. A number of urine tests for bladder cancer are being evaluated, including BTA stat, NMP22, telomerase, UBC marker and Immunocyst. So far, none of these tests have sufficient sensitivity and specificity to be useful in screening. Some of them may have a part to play in follow-up of patients with known disease, and could theoretically allow more frequent and non-invasive monitoring for recurrence.

Prompt presentation. All too often, patients with bladder tumors experience considerable delay in diagnosis. This may be because the patient does not report an isolated episode of hematuria, because the primary care physician ignores non-persistent hematuria, or because of delays imposed by the healthcare system.

It is vital that patients and their primary care physicians are aware that bleeding from a bladder tumor may be intermittent, and that even a single episode of hematuria must be investigated. The process of hospital referral can be accelerated by establishing one-stop hematuria clinics.

The increasing weight of evidence that delay in treatment adversely affects outcome is prompting strenuous efforts to reduce such delays, though it has to be said that in the UK at least there is still some way to go.

Improvements in management of high-risk superficial disease

Although high-risk superficial disease represents only a small proportion of new cases of bladder cancer (10–20% in most series), it is important because, if well treated, it can be controlled, but if inadequately treated, it can rapidly become invasive and metastasize.

Increasing awareness of the lethal potential of high-risk superficial bladder cancer and concomitant action will result in improved survival. Treatment with BCG is now accepted as best practice, and the need for early cystectomy for BCG-resistant disease is more commonly recognized.

Improvements in existing treatments

Advances have been made recently in defining the risk of local recurrence and progression to invasive disease faced by patients with superficial disease. By considering factors such as tumor grade, number of tumors at presentation, presence of associated CIS and pattern of recurrence, patients can be divided into low-, intermediate- and high-risk groups. This allows a reduction in the frequency of cystoscopies in the low-risk group, and early introduction of intravesical chemotherapy with closer follow-up of those at greater risk. Recognition of the life-threatening nature of extensive CIS and grade 3 T1 tumors has brought about a more aggressive treatment policy, with early radical surgery offered if intravesical BCG or appropriate intravesical chemotherapy fails to eradicate the tumor.

Additional information about the potential for progression in patients with superficial disease may be available by studying p53 expression. This gene codes for a tumor suppressor, and p53 mutation is associated with an increased risk of invasion; thus, expression levels may identify those patients needing BCG or early cystectomy.

Earlier recourse to cystectomy or radiotherapy in patients with muscle-invasive disease should improve survival, and patient and surgeon reluctance to consider radical treatment will be reduced by the availability of techniques that avoid urostomy. There is evidence that more meticulous node dissection in cystectomy improves survival, but changes in surgical practice will have only a small overall influence on survival.

Ongoing studies are reevaluating the role of adjuvant chemotherapy, and a modest survival benefit is expected. In this context, new, less toxic combinations such as gemcitabine and cisplatin may be used.

Chemoradiation is another treatment option under assessment. Studies are in progress of the response of tumors to a course of chemotherapy, in which responders complete the course and also receive radiotherapy, while non-responders undergo cystectomy. This approach may allow bladder preservation in some patients without compromising the chance of cure in patients whose tumor is not chemo- or radiosensitive.

The increasing trend for patients to be managed by a multidisciplinary team should mean that all patients are offered the best available therapy.

Development of new treatments

The search for effective systemic cytotoxic therapy continues, with new drugs and drug combinations being evaluated. If chemotherapy can achieve a significant complete response rate in advanced disease, the hope of effective adjuvant therapy in early disease might be realized.

The use of drugs to counter tumor resistance to intravesical chemotherapy by sensitizing the tumor promises to improve the response of superficial disease, but has yet to be evaluated in a clinical setting.

The treatment of superficial disease with photodynamic therapy is being explored. Certain drugs, given systemically or intravesically, are taken up by tumor cells. When exposed to laser light of a specific wavelength, the drugs have a cytotoxic effect on the tumor cells. Clinical trials of this form of therapy are at an early stage.

The evaluation of genetic markers of the potential for invasion may help identify those patients with superficial disease at the greatest risk of progression, who would therefore benefit from more aggressive treatment.

Better understanding of the mechanism of invasion and metastasis at a molecular level may bring a new range of therapies. Knowledge of the role of angiogenesis in establishing metastases, for example, has led to the development of angiogenesis inhibitors, which are now being evaluated experimentally. The nature of cell-to-cell adhesion, telomerase activity and matrix metalloproteinases are all subjects of research, and translation into human trials is at an early stage. Gene therapy is being explored, including targeting tumor suppressor genes such as p53, angiogenesis factors, immunomodulation and prodrug activation therapy. Use of these treatments in metastatic disease is complicated by the difficulties of direct access to the tumor to be treated. However, the convenience of intravesical administration for local disease makes bladder cancer an ideal target for some of these therapies.

At present, there is little prospect of preventing bladder cancer. Metastatic disease is seldom cured by available treatments. The best immediate options for improvement are therefore early diagnosis and better recognition of the life-threatening nature of high-grade superficial disease.

Useful resources

National Cancer Institute (USA)
Tel: 1 800 422 6237
(Mon–Fri 9 AM – 4:30 PM)
cancergovstaff@mail.nih.gov
www.cancer.gov/cancertopics/types/
bladder

Cancerhelp UK
Cancer Information Department
Cancer Research UK
PO Box 123
Lincoln's Inn Fields
London WC2A 3PX
www.cancerhelp.org.uk

The Continence Foundation
307 Hatton Square
16 Baldwins Gardens
London EC1N 7RJ
Tel: 0845 345 0165
(Mon–Fri 9:30 AM – 1 PM)
continence-help@dial.pipex.com
www.continence-foundation.org.uk

The Urostomy Association (UK)
Central Office
18 Foxglove Avenue
Uttoxeter
Staffordshire ST14 8UN
secretary.ua@classmail.co.uk
www.uagbi.org

American Cancer Society
Bladder cancer pages
www.cancer.org/docroot/lrn/
lrn_0.asp

Cancer Link USA
Bladder cancer pages
www.cancerlinksusa.com/bladder/
index.asp

CancerBACUP
Bladder cancer pages
www.cancerbacup.org.uk/
cancertype/bladder

Cancer Research UK
Bladder cancer site
www.cancerhelp.org.uk/help/
default.asp?page=2680

Cancer Index
www.cancerindex.org/clinks3d.htm

Index

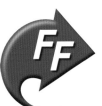

Imagine if every time you wanted to know something you knew where to look...

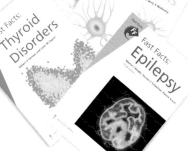

Over one million copies sold

- Written by world experts
- Concise and practical
- Up to date
- Designed for ease of reading and reference
- Copiously illustrated with useful photographs, diagrams and charts.

Our aim is to make *Fast Facts* the world's most respected medical handbook series. Feedback on how to make titles even more useful is always welcome (feedback@fastfacts.com).

More than 70 *Fast Facts* titles, including:

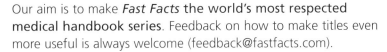

Asthma	Inflammatory Bowel Disease (second edition)
Benign Gynecological Disease (second edition)	Irritable Bowel Syndrome (second edition)
Benign Prostatic Hyperplasia (fifth edition)	Menopause (second edition)
Bipolar Disorder	Minor Surgery
Bleeding Disorders	Multiple Sclerosis (second edition)
Brain Tumors	Obstructive Sleep Apnea
Breast Cancer (third edition)	Osteoporosis (fourth edition)
Chronic Obstructive Pulmonary Disease	Parkinson's Disease
Colorectal Cancer (second edition)	Prostate Cancer (fourth edition)
Contraception (second edition)	Psoriasis (second edition)
Dementia	Renal Disorders
Depression (second edition)	Respiratory Tract Infection (second edition)
Dyspepsia (second edition)	Rheumatoid Arthritis
Eczema and Contact Dermatitis	Schizophrenia (second edition)
Endometriosis (second edition)	Sexual Dysfunction
Epilepsy (third edition)	Sexually Transmitted Infections
Erectile Dysfunction (third edition)	Skin Cancer
Gynecological Oncology	Smoking Cessation
Headaches (second edition)	Soft Tissue Rheumatology
Hyperlipidemia (third edition)	Thyroid Disorders
Hypertension (second edition)	Urinary Stones

Orders

To order via the website, or to find regional distributors, please go to www.fastfacts.com

For telephone orders, please call +44 (0)1752 202301 (Europe), 1 800 247 6553 (USA, toll free) or +1 419 281 1802 (Americas)

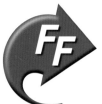

Imagine if every time
you wanted to know something
you knew where to look...

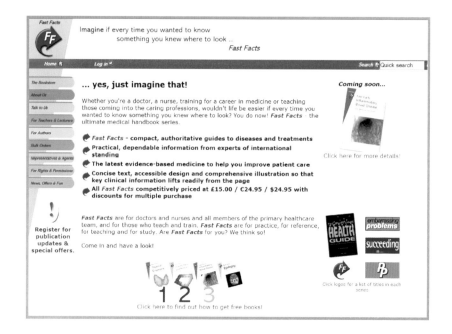

... **you do now!**

www.fastfacts.com